The
Cheat to Lose
Diet

Joel Marion, CISSN, NSCA-CPT
with recipes by John Berardi, Ph.D.,
author of *The Metabolism Advantage*

CROWN PUBLISHERS
NEW YORK

The Cheat to Lose Diet

Cheat BIG with the Foods You Love,
Lose Fat Faster Than Ever Before,
and Enjoy Keeping It Off!

The information presented in this work is in no way intended as medical advice or as a substitute for medical counseling. The information should be used in conjunction with the guidance and care of your physician. Consult your physician before beginning this program as you would any weight-loss or weight-maintenance program. Your physician should be aware of all medical conditions that you may have as well as the medications and supplements you are taking. As with any weight-loss plan, the information here should not be used by patients on dialysis or by pregnant or nursing mothers. The author and the publisher expressly disclaim responsibility for any adverse effects that may result from the use or application of the information contained in this book.

Copyright © 2007 by Joel Marion

Recipes © 2007 by John Berardi

All rights reserved.

Published in the United States by Crown Publishers, an imprint of the Crown Publishing Group, a division of Random House, Inc., New York.

www.crownpublishing.com

Crown is a trademark and the Crown colophon is a registered trademark of Random House, Inc.

Library of Congress Cataloging-in-Publication Data

Marion, Joel.

The cheat to lose diet: cheat big with the foods you love, lose fat faster than ever before, and enjoy keeping it off! / Joel Marion.—1st ed.

Includes index.

1. Weight loss.   2. Weight loss—Psychological aspects.   I. Title.

RM222.2.M3575 2007

613.2'5—dc22   2006037006

ISBN 978-0-307-35224-8

Printed in the United States of America

Design by Chris Welch

1 3 5 7 9 10 8 6 4 2

First Edition

For my brothers, Phil and Gary,
whose undying friendship, support,
and belief have seen me through
to this moment.
Here's to JPG's.

Acknowledgments

First and foremost, thanks be to God, for without you and your many blessings this book would never have come to fruition.

To my agent, Mel Berger—from day one, you have believed in this project as much as I have. Moreover, you have believed in me. It's an honor to be represented by you.

To my editor, my friend, my partner, Heather Jackson—the time and effort you have expended working with me, together, through all the ups, downs, ins, and outs of this book are more than anyone could ask for. You are tremendous.

To my friend and colleague Dr. John Berardi—as I began my career in health and fitness, you took me under your wing. Your encouragement and words of wisdom helped to mold me as a young author, and now, years later, it's been my pleasure to have you as part of this project.

To Dr. Derek LeJeune, who has so graciously provided the foreword to this book—your recognition of my hard work is greatly appreciated, and even more so are the insights you have shared with me throughout the last five years. Thank you.

To the team at Crown—if I've ever experienced love at first sight, it was at our initial NYC meeting. Within fifteen minutes it was clear that we had a shared vision, and I knew there were no better hands to place this book into. I'm excited to be working with you and am excited to explore the future—together.

To Body-for-Life Challenge directors Shane Thomas and Marc Bennett—your belief in me back in 2001 propelled me to further fulfill my utmost potential. Moreover, it has had the most rewarding compound effect, with your initial belief fueling the impact I've been so fortunate to have on lives all around the world. For that, I am indebted to you.

To my teachers through the years, specifically Bob Newman, David Boudwin, Chris Abiuso, Morris "Coach" Loveland, Sherrie Gumienny, and Art Chilakos—your impact on me, my dreams, and my ambitions is greater than you know. You instilled passion within me. You are my mentors, and I'm extremely lucky to be a product of your influence.

To Phil, Beth, Gary, and Lindsay—some will go a lifetime never experiencing the bond and closeness of a friendship like the one we share. You've been with me through everything, every step of the way, and without question are my driving force.

To my parents—you have watched me develop and grow under your direction. I only hope I've made and will continue to make you proud. You did a great job.

And finally, to you, the reader—without you I'd have no one to share my passion with. Thank you for your faith—in this book, but more important, in yourself. This program, in all its practicality, is for you, your health—*your life*. You can and will succeed.

Contents

Foreword

As an M.D., I believe a diet must meet three criteria for me to either use it myself or recommend it to my patients. First and foremost, it must be scientifically and medically sound. Second, it must be healthful. And finally, the approach must be one that is realistic for the average American to follow. I can emphatically say *The Cheat to Lose Diet* by Joel Marion has accomplished all three, and to a degree unmatched by its predecessors.

Before elaborating on the above, allow me to share some personal experience. I am not simply a doctor loosely lending my stamp of approval to the latest diet trend; no, my recommendation carries much more weight than that. I have known Joel for more than five years, and the two of us would often discuss his developing theories on the use of dietary cheating to accelerate fat loss. In 2003, when he first cemented his theories to create the Cheat to Lose approach, I was one of the first to put the program to the test and experience just how effortless dieting and fat loss was always meant to be. Yes, you heard correctly—a medical doctor turned to a fitness professional for dietary guidance. Sure, as a physician, I had extensive knowledge of healthy nutritional habits, but Joel's approach was intriguing, exciting, and based on the most recent, cutting-edge medical literature. Not only that, but despite being a doctor, I'm also human and share with every American a love for good food. With Cheat to Lose, I knew I'd be able to achieve and maintain optimal health while still consuming all of my favorite foods. This made Joel's the first and only diet I've ever found to be personally appealing in addition to medically interesting.

And while I'm on the topic of credentials, allow me to take a minute to speak on behalf of Joel's credibility. I do not know of *anyone* who has put more time, effort, enthusiasm, and passion into ensuring the validity and effectiveness of the approach he advocates. If there is anyone qualified to write a book on health and weight loss, it's Joel. In addition to practicing what he preaches and making such dramatic improvements to his own physique, Joel has spent literally years of his life sorting through the available research. Because of his unbiased review of the literature, Joel is more qualified than some others in the medical community who continually look to only one side of the coin. Furthermore, Joel brings to the table something that very few others do—real-life experience with hundreds of individuals from all over the world. In addition to being so strongly medically rooted, Joel's theories have been refined and balanced by the experiences of his clients. This does wonders for the credibility and efficacy of Joel's methods by bridging the gap between scientific theory and real-world practice—a gap so many other approaches and authors leave untouched.

Going back to my initial three criteria, the theories and assertions of *The Cheat to Lose Diet* are extensively supported by the medical literature. The research Joel has provided represents some of the most forward-looking studies and comprehensive review papers to date on the topics of nutritional practices and their resulting metabolic and hormonal responses. With more than three hundred references in the book, Joel has certainly done his homework to ensure that his recommendations are both scientifically and medically sound. And what's more, he is able to clearly communicate this research in a way that makes absorbing the science an easy task that is both fun and interesting.

Second, *The Cheat to Lose Diet* provides a healthy approach to weight loss. In contrast to so many other diets that employ radical, unnecessary methods and extreme limitation to achieve results that are often very short-lived, Cheat to Lose limits nothing and concentrates on long-term, maintainable weight loss. Unlike other popular diets, you will not heavily restrict carbohydrate or fat intake; instead, you will enjoy literally every carbohydrate you can think of, from fruits and vegetables to breads and pastas. You'll learn the importance of fat in the diet and learn how to choose healthy fats. Throughout the course of Cheat to Lose, you will take measures to maintain a healthy metabolic rate, so that once you've reached your goal weight, you'll be able to remain at that weight for a long time to come.

Lastly, *The Cheat to Lose Diet* is practical in its approach— perhaps the most important of the three criteria. You will not feel deprived. You will not experience intense cravings. But you *will* enjoy the widest selection of foods of any diet currently available. Moreover, you are *required* to cheat. For the average American, that's as realistic and practical as it gets.

To summarize, *The Cheat to Lose Diet* is a true gold mine of nutritional insight and practical dietary information. There isn't an easier, more comprehensive plan out there that makes more sense, both physically and psychologically. If you're looking for a way to lose weight and keep it off, this is it. And although this is unusual when speaking of dieting, I'm confident that you'll actually enjoy the process immensely in addition to the extraordinary results—just as I have.

In health,

Derek LeJeune, M.D.

Dr. LeJeune received his medical degree from Louisiana State University Health Sciences Center in New Orleans. He is a practicing physician in the Dallas, Texas, area, where he lives with his wife, Laurie.

PART I

The Cheat to Lose Program

art I is dedicated to the Cheat to Lose Program. In this section, we'll dive headfirst into the discovery, development, science, and specifics of the Cheat to Lose Diet. As the beginning chapters come to a close, you will understand completely why regular dietary cheating is the solution to the many problems most all commercial diets create. Furthermore, the remaining chapters of Part I will equip you with every bit of knowledge necessary to successfully implement and gain fantastic results from the Cheat to Lose approach. In chapter 7, I'll also outline a true cheater's exercise program—the CTL Cardio Solution—to complement the dietary information provided and to ensure that you're achieving the fastest possible results. Cheating with the intent to lose—it's no longer a paradox.

Prior to Cheat to Lose, the longest I lasted on any sort of diet was about a month. That's when the cravings would really start to kick in, and I'd fall victim to them every time. I just didn't have the willpower it took to stay on a diet, or at least that's what I thought. Then I read about Joel's Cheat to Lose Diet and how he actually encourages dieters to cheat on a regular basis. I was definitely a pro at cheating, so I decided to give it a try. The weekly planned cheating of the Cheat to Lose Diet had me cheating with a purpose instead of being emotionally distraught by random screwups. Finally, I found a diet that I can actually stick to. Six months later, I've kept off the 20 pounds of fat I lost (going from 127 to 107 at 5'2") and love the energy I have each day to spend on my kids.

Christina J.
Fredericksburg,
Virginia

In eight weeks, I cheated to lose 18 pounds and 14½ inches! I'm now fitting back into jeans I wore almost ten years ago in high school, and there's no way I would have been able to do it without the Cheat to Lose Diet. I've never been able to stick to a diet because I've never been able to week after week deprive myself of my most favorite foods; well, with the Cheat to Lose Diet, I didn't have to! I've gotten so many compliments from friends and family members, and even just recently bought some new sexy clothing to wear out. My boyfriend is proud of me, I'm proud of myself, and I'm both look-ing and feeling great!

Erin M.
Arlington, Virginia

We decided to do the Cheat to Lose Diet as a family—and it's been a wonderful experience all around. In only eight weeks' time, I lost over 5 percent body fat, my wife was finally able to rid herself of those last 10 pounds she had been struggling to lose (and has kept them off), and my sixteen-year-old son is now more than 20 pounds lighter. To-gether, as a family, we have encouraged each other and pulled each other through—but we couldn't have done it without an approach like the Cheat to Lose Diet. With other diets, we'd fail, as they limited too many things. With the Cheat to Lose Diet, we learned how to enjoy all types of foods in their right time and place—including things like pizza and ice cream. The Cheat Day was an excellent motivator for us, as it encouraged good behavior to be rewarded later. Because of CTL, my family is now enjoying eating, looking, and being healthier. Addition-ally, there is no value that can be put on the compliments we receive from friends and other family members when they see us. We're very proud of our accomplishments and thankful for a program such as Cheat to Lose that has made those accomplishments both achievable and maintainable.

The Clark family
Benton, Kentucky

A Cheater's Introduction

The Cheat to Lose Diet has completely changed my life. I am 50 pounds lighter and have lost more than 10 inches around my waist—and I'm still going. I have confidence again. I have a feeling that I will be there for my son when he grows up. I have self-respect again, and I feel I have regained respect from others. There is no aspect of my life that has not changed for the better since I started the Cheat to Lose Diet. I honestly believe if I had not discovered Cheat to Lose, I would be over 300 pounds right now, depressed, not doing well at work, and not being a great dad to my son. Instead, I am happy, healthy, full of energy, and confident. I have been hiking with my more-than-25-pound son on my back, going up trails I could not have done a year ago with no additional weight. I am doing things on the tennis court and the hockey rink that I have not been able to do for years. I am even thinking of participating in a triathlon this upcoming year. My life has changed, as well as my lifestyle and my overall level of happiness and success. Without this approach, I would never be able to stick to a diet, and my past is proof of just that. For me, this is not a diet; it is a way of life. Thank you, Cheat to Lose!

Timm B.

Denver, Colorado

'm absolutely thrilled that you are reading this book! Why am I thrilled? Because I know the information contained in the next nine chapters is going to help you change your habits, your body, and ultimately your *life*. In the pages to follow, I am going to unveil to you a diet that couldn't be any easier to follow but at the same time is going to prove to be the most effective diet you have ever tried. Sound like an oxymoron? Maybe before, but with the Cheat to Lose Diet, it's reality. You will not be deprived; you will eat the foods you crave, and you will lose fat faster than ever before. This diet is one that anyone, and I mean *anyone,* can have success with. You may be someone who has tried every diet under the sun to no avail, but as sure as you are reading this book, that is going to change—big-time.

Ingredients for Success

It has been said that a diet is only as effective as the number of people who can stick with it, and wow, that statement couldn't be any more true! While many of today's premier diets look enticing on paper, their success rates, or the number of people who actually follow through on them for any length of time, leave much to be desired. A diet can be great in theory, but if it's not practical for the average person to follow in the short and long term, it's not worth a whole lot.

On the opposite end of the spectrum are oversimplified, dumbed-down diets making claims while rarely delivering on them. These fad diets are temporarily embraced by the media and general public with exaggerated zeal because of their extreme simplicity and alluring promises. Unfortunately, the popularity of such diets is short-lived, as they continually fail to produce lasting results. Albert Einstein once said, "Everything should be made as simple as possible, but not simpler." While the diets in question are initially appealing, they'll never stand the test of time when sacrificing effectiveness for simplicity. For a diet to be valuable, it needs to be both practical *and* effective, and that's exactly what the Cheat to Lose Diet is.

This Diet Was Developed by a Screwup

And that's the truth, folks. If I were perfect, I never would have discovered how effective an approach like Cheat to Lose could be; I never would have developed this diet, and I never would have written this book. You see, in the early months of 2002, I was on a mission—a mission to be in the best physical shape of my life. Extremely determined, I formulated my plan of attack and made up my mind that there would be no deviating from it—and that meant no pizza, ice cream, potato chips, cookies (oh, my beloved chocolate chip cookies), candy, or any other food that wasn't on my preapproved list. "Absolutely *no* cheating!" I told myself. I knew it wouldn't be easy, but I also knew it was what I had to do to make my goals reality. Or so I thought then.

No more than a month into the diet, I hit a wall—a big wall— and over the course of the next few weeks neither the scale nor the image in the mirror seemed to change. I became discouraged, and given my relatively limited knowledge of the body's natural feedback systems at the time, I had no clue as to why my progress had come to such a screeching halt despite my religious adherence to the program.

Then I went to a party hosted by a friend of mine that included fun, games, and plenty of good food. Now, anyone who knows me will attest to the fact that I love to eat. It's common knowledge that to ensure that enough food is present, I need to be counted as three guests—minimum. And the fact that I wasn't eating *anything* at the party concerned quite a few individuals. From the moment I walked in the door, I was surrounded by food. Within ten minutes, I had been offered something to eat at least half a dozen times. After hearing me repeatedly (albeit reluctantly) utter the words "No, thank you," people began to ask why I wasn't eating. I told them I was dieting, and after dealing with the usual "Come on, live a little!" response, I continued to socialize. About a half hour later, I made the mistake of walking into the kitchen. Everything smelled *so* good—pasta, meatballs, Italian bread and pastries, crackers, cookies, chips, and cake. Before I knew it, I was living up to my reputation, devouring plate after plate of pasta, meatballs, warm Italian bread, desserts, and just about anything else I could get my hands on.

When I got home from the party, I immediately sprawled out on the couch and let the insulin and serotonin rush I'd triggered do its thing. I slept like a baby. Unfortunately, when I woke up, I did so in a cloud of guilt. I felt like a failure. I'd broken the plan. Instead of sucking it up when things got difficult, I'd given in and become careless. Still, I had goals to reach, and I couldn't let my screwup keep me down.

Over the course of the next few days, I got back on track with my diet and exercise program and was doing quite well. But it wasn't very long until I was tempted again. No more than a week later, I walked in the door from a long day of work to find two freshly baked pizzas sitting on the kitchen table. Man, was it ever the wrong time for something like this to happen; I hadn't eaten in hours and was starving.

I figured a slice or two wouldn't kill me, but that "slice or two" turned into half a pie, then six slices, and eventually I put the finishing touches on an entire large pizza. At that point, I became pretty liberal about what I ate for the rest of the evening. I figured the night was already lost, so why not enjoy it and then start fresh tomorrow? Needless to say, I splurged into the wee hours of the morning, running up quite an impressive calorie total along the way. Screwup number two was now a page in the history books.

Once again, I resumed my program in hopes of making up the lost ground. In just a few short days, the initial bloat and water retention resulting from my massive feast had faded, and surprisingly, I actually appeared to be leaner than I'd been two weeks before. This made me understandably curious, so I decided to step on the scale (something I had been adamantly avoiding) to find out what was happening. I was down 3 pounds. How in the world had the most undedicated, screwed-up two weeks of my dietary life pulled me out of a major fat-loss rut and result in a 3-pound loss of flab?

I can't say that I was tremendously surprised by what had just happened. In the past, when attempting to shed unwanted body fat, I'd allowed myself to periodically have a day in which I didn't take my diet so seriously. Provided that I immediately got back to business with my program, the approach worked fairly well. At times, however, I would cut out any and all cheating with the intention of accelerating my progress or breaking through a fat-loss plateau. Unfortunately, that never really worked. Every time I tried to be extremely strict with my diet, it didn't accelerate much of anything, and oftentimes progress seemed even slower. I blamed the stalled fat loss on something else, though (not exercising enough, not limiting calories enough, etc.), instead of making a correlation between eliminating the cheating and my lack of results. Why, after experiencing this trend, had I failed to make the connection? I think the answer is simple: the concept that cheating could be beneficial seemed to defy logical reasoning. It just doesn't seem to make sense. Luckily, though, our bodies are a lot smarter than we are.

At this point, I was convinced that what I had experienced was more than just coincidence, so I started browsing through various peer-reviewed journals and databases and taking a deeper look into what happens in our bodies when we diet and what happens when we overeat. What I discovered through searching the medical literature proved to be very interesting. I continued to read, learn, and experiment with both myself and my clients during the next several months. To say that the results people were experiencing were intriguing would be a serious understatement. People absolutely loved the effectiveness and practicality of the approach I had developed. Cheat to Lose was helping individuals achieve things they had never been able to do before—and that was exciting!

Later that year, I wrote my first article on the subject, and I have since written a myriad more. Literally thousands of individuals have benefited from the approach to date, and every client's experience has helped me to perfect the setup further. Now, more than three years later, I can say with confidence that I have been able to bridge the gap between the science and what actually happens in the real world and have pinned down the most effective way to incorporate periodic cheating into a diet plan to yield the fastest, least painful results you have ever experienced. This finalized approach, while used by many of my individual clients, has also been extensively researched via several large participant test groups. Throughout this book, many of these clients and test subjects will share with you their personal experiences on the Cheat to Lose Diet—experiences that I'm certain will both challenge and motivate you as you read them.

You Have the Power

Having said that, the Cheat to Lose Diet will still require a degree of effort on your part. Yes, you will eat the foods you love without feeling guilty (because you will learn that when it is done properly, doing so can actually accelerate your progress), and yes, you will find this diet much easier to adhere to than any other you have ever tried, but anytime you embark on a mission to change, you can rest assured that there will be times when your self-control, willpower, and determination are put to the test. During these times, you will be tempted to throw in the towel (temporarily or permanently) and revert to old habits. And whether or not you are able to persevere through such times is going to determine the amount of success you have with this diet.

From those who read this book, three groups will emerge. There will be those who read the book and find it interesting but take no action. For these individuals, the book serves as a means of entertainment, but unfortunately, that's about all. While their intentions may be to "someday" start the diet, that day is and always will be tomorrow. Others will read the book and quickly begin the diet with great excitement. After only a few short weeks (or even days), however, when the initial enthusiasm has faded and the challenges of exchanging old habits for new ones surface, they will renege on their commitment. They'll give up on the program, their goals, and themselves. Then there are those readers who will be inspired to change, and will decide that they're going to do whatever it takes. These individuals will realize that the Cheat to Lose Diet is a diet that they *can* have success with. Despite being faced with challenges, they will triumph. Sure, they may slip, but if they do, they'll get up, brush themselves off, and continue in the direction of their goals. Which group will you belong to? Will you choose to make a commitment to yourself and stick with it? Will you choose to change your body? Will you choose to take charge of your health? Or will you allow the opportunity to change slip through your fingers?

This book will give you a recipe for success—a proven, scientific method to achieve fast, relatively painless fat loss—but only *you* can bring value to the words on these pages. The question you have to ask yourself is "How serious am I about achieving my goals?" Whatever your goals, there is no doubt in my mind that the Cheat to Lose Diet will prove to be the most effective, enjoyable means to achieving them—period.

What Makes the Cheat to Lose Diet Different?

The Cheat to Lose Diet has completely changed the way I look at dieting. I had always experienced the quick plateau Joel talks about when trying to be extremely strict with my diet, and now I know why—I was fighting a losing battle against my own body! Restriction, restriction, restriction—all leading nowhere. Now when I indulge, I do so without apprehension because not only do I understand how it will accelerate fat loss, I see the results. The setup of Cheat to Lose has helped me lose fat and gain confidence, all while enjoying life to its fullest. Denying oneself the finer things in life, one of which is certainly good food, really is no way to live. This is a long-term approach to weight management.

Barry M.

Ireland

Dieting doesn't mean restriction anymore. I always looked at dieting as a thing of denial, but on the Cheat to Lose Diet, there are just too many options when it comes to the food I'm able to eat for me to feel even the least bit deprived. I've never experienced such freedom while dieting ever before. It amazes me to be eating like this and losing more weight than I was when being restrictive and eating so little. In ten weeks, I have lost 33 pounds of pure fat. That's incredible. My energy is through the roof. This experience has spilled over to every area of my life—I'm now more passionate than ever about achieving my work- and family-related goals, and am working toward them with much improved confidence and health.

Dave A.

Tyrone, Northern Ireland

To me, diet is the most offensive of any four-letter word. It implies restriction, deprivation, and struggle—all for very little in the end most times. The Cheat to Lose Diet is none of these things. Instead, it's fun, it's full of choices and plenty of good food, and most important, it works. I was coming off a back injury and very little physical activity for over a month, and Cheat to Lose helped me easily lose over 20 pounds of unwanted body fat in less than three months' time. I'm happier, my wife is happier, and my life in general has benefited greatly because of it—that's a true reward.

Mustafa B.

Japan

I was thin until I was thirty and had my first child. The first few years with her, I didn't think about the weight because I was so busy having fun. That said, being heavy had started to become more bothersome to me over the last several years. I wanted my cute figure back, but for a long time getting it back was no easy task. Then I learned about Cheat to Lose. With Joel's diet, I learned how to lose body fat while still consuming my favorite foods on a weekly basis. The science behind the program made so much sense, and before long, my reflection in the mirror was backing up the science with real-world results. Ironically, I'd noticed the phenomenon of cheating and then subsequently losing weight previously, but I'd had no idea how or when to use the tactic. Cheat to Lose showed me how. This is an easy, fun way to lose weight that I can see myself sticking with for a long time to come. And the best part is that the first place the weight came off was my belly and hips—my most troublesome areas after pregnancy!

Heather C.

Richland Hills, Texas

Diet books are a dime a dozen. Walk into a bookstore and you'll find more of them than you can count; attend a family get-together and without a doubt the talk of the evening will be the various diets family members are currently embarking on; surf through a night of television talk shows and news broadcasts and within one of the lineups there is sure to be an author promoting his or her guide to weight loss. And now you're being presented with yet another one—another book, another diet, another method for losing that unwanted flab surrounding your midsection. But Cheat to Lose isn't just another diet. No, Cheat to Lose distinguishes itself by being the only diet specifically designed to work *with* your body's natural feedback systems, both psychological and physiological, instead of against them. This means less frustration, faster results, and overall a much more bearable diet.

Arghhhhhhhh!

Ever feel this way? Or maybe a better question is: ever been on a diet? Why is dieting so psychologically draining? Well, for one, it requires change in a major area of our lives—the way we eat— and for most of us, change is a very uncomfortable thing. Changing old habits and forming new ones is never an easy task; however, with dieting, it becomes exceedingly difficult given all of the physiological adaptations that occur (which we will soon discuss).

Consider what happens psychologically when you go on a diet. Almost immediately you are faced with an array of cravings. Just the sight or smell of food adds to your already present hunger pangs. You find yourself craving foods that normally you have no desire to eat. Every time you come in contact with an off-limits food item—whether on a television commercial, in a magazine, or physically right in front of you—the battle begins. Do you give in to the temptation to experience immediate pleasure, only to be swarmed by overwhelming guilt shortly after? Or do you stick it out and allow the anxiety to increase with every day? It seems like a lose-lose situation—and it is.

And what if you're not making as much progress as you had hoped? What if you're seemingly doing everything right and the scale just isn't moving? Feelings of frustration, discouragement, and even depression emerge, making you even more inclined to break your diet. I mean, who wants to sacrifice without being rewarded? At least when you bite into a chocolate chip cookie, the taste is satisfying. But working hard to reap no return on investment, well, that's just no good at all.

Dieting is a mental battle from day one. But in reality, all of these things that we experience psychologically while reducing calories are the result of a bigger problem—your body's physio-logical response to your fat-loss attempts.

Going Head-to-Head with Nature

What most people don't realize is that the very concept of dieting is in direct opposition to the desired outcomes of going on a diet! As soon as you begin to restrict calories your brain sends out a number of hormonal signals informing the body to put the brakes on metabolism and to hold on to that stubborn fat you're trying to kiss good-bye. For this to make any kind of sense, we need to think back to primitive times. In such times, it was not very likely that you would come across a physique-conscious individual; peo-ple of this time period had more important things to worry about than their reflection in the nearest stream—things like surviving. In order to survive, one had to eat. Unfortunately, driving to the local supermarket and picking up a prepackaged meal for dinner wasn't an option back then, so to nourish themselves, our ances-tors had to hunt for food. Even when food was more accessible in the warmer months, there were still periods of time when provi-sions were scarce. For instance, a family might feast on a kill for a few days and then go a few days with very little food while out searching for more game. On a larger scale, during the winter months food was in short supply, leaving our ancestors in an un-derfed state for months at a time. During these times, the body responds with its natural defense against starvation—"bad" hor-mones, fat-storage enzymes, and hunger all increase while "good" hormones, metabolism, and fat-burning enzymes take a dive. In other words, as a survival mechanism, the body does everything it can to hold on to body fat.

Today, we are faced with a similar response each and every time we go on a reduced-calorie diet. Dieting, although planned, is just a lesser degree of starvation. Your body isn't aware of your hopes for six-pack abs or your efforts toward buns of steel; all it knows is that you are consuming fewer calories than you need, and to the brain, that's a big red flag.

When a stressor is present, the body's job, without exception, is to take the necessary precautions to keep you alive. This is a great thing when you're infected with a virus or foreign bacterium, or if you're stranded on a desolate island somewhere; however, this type of response isn't so wonderful when you're trying to chip away at the ol' love handles. And the longer you remain in a caloric deficit, the more pronounced the response becomes. Before you know it, fat is coming off extremely slowly, and despite your dieting efforts the scale doesn't seem to be moving and your appearance doesn't seem to be changing.

One of the major players in this whole chain of events is the hormone leptin, named after the Greek word *leptos*, meaning "thin." Granted, there are many other hormones that play a role and reactions that take place in the regulation of body weight and metabolism, but for the purpose of this book, leptin is the main one we need to understand. You may or may not have heard of leptin, but since its discovery in the mid-1990s much research has been conducted on the hormone, and now, over a decade later, we are finally beginning to understand the metabolic adaptations that occur in our bodies while dieting.

Leptin is a hormone produced by and released from fat cells; it floats around in the blood and communicates your "starvation status" to the brain. Under normal conditions, leptin is abundant and the brain receives the message that everything is normal. When an individual is very thin and/or not consuming enough food, leptin blood levels are low and consequently that red flag message is sent to the brain. These blood levels are controlled by two factors. One is the amount of body fat you are carrying. Since leptin's origin is the fat cell, it only makes sense that there is a direct, linear relationship between leptin and body fat. This is of particular importance when dieting because as fat is lost, baseline leptin levels decrease. Less fat = less leptin. Less leptin = red flag message to the brain.

The second factor impacting blood leptin levels is the amount of food you are taking in, or your caloric intake. The same direct, linear relationship that exists between leptin and body fat exists between leptin and the amount of food you eat. It was originally thought that leptin levels were mediated solely by body fat levels, but more recent studies have shown that caloric intake affects leptin levels independent of fat mass. One particular study noted that leptin levels of dieters decreased by an average of approximately 50 percent after only one week of caloric restriction; however, subjects only lost a very small amount of body fat during this time (certainly not anywhere close to 50 percent). In other words, if someone is significantly overweight but eating very little, he or she will still suffer from low leptin concentrations and the associated metabolic disadvantages. Caloric restriction = low leptin levels. Low leptin levels = red flag message to the brain.

Let's talk about what happens when the brain receives this red flag message. After receiving the memo, the brain responds by sending out various regulatory signals to the rest of the body, causing quite a few adverse reactions (from a dieting standpoint) to occur. Levels of thyroid hormones, which play a major role in the regulation of metabolism and energy expenditure, significantly decline. Overall metabolic rate and twenty-four-hour energy expenditure plummet to balance caloric output with caloric intake so as to preserve fat mass. Serum cortisol, a stress hormone largely responsible for abdominal fat storage and muscle wasting, skyrockets as leptin levels fall. And then, concentrations of ghrelin, an appetite-regulating hormone produced in the stomach, increase dramatically, causing intense hunger and cravings.

No wonder succeeding on a diet is so difficult—we're fighting a losing battle against our own bodies! As soon as we drop calories, leptin levels quickly fall and continue to gradually decrease. Then, for every pound of progress we make, our bodies fight back by dropping leptin even lower, which in turn tightens the clamps on fat burning. The more fat we lose, the more difficult it becomes to keep losing fat.

Briefly going back to the psychology of it all, think of how demoralizing this is for us as dieters. Here we are striving to do all we can to change, yet we're not making progress. As if change weren't hard enough as it is, now we have our own bodies prohibiting us from doing so despite our effort.

What can be done to combat these adaptations and to keep the fat-burning furnace stoked? If falling leptin levels are responsible for metabolic shutdown and slowed fat loss, then why not just supplement with a synthetic leptin product (i.e., leptin in a bottle or something similar)? Unfortunately, it's not quite that easy, and leptin researcher Lyle McDonald notes several reasons why. First, leptin is a protein-based hormone, so it can't be taken orally. Therefore, the method of administration would have to be injection. This puts the nutritional supplement industry out of the race, as any supplement/medication that needs to be injected can only be obtained with a prescription (although, believe it or not, there are a few diet pill products out there claiming to contain leptin, which are obvious scams for the reason just mentioned). That leaves things up to the pharmaceutical industry; however, it isn't all that interested, for a few reasons. First, there is the injection issue. An injectable medication, simply because it requires one to plunge a needle deep into the skin daily, wouldn't exactly be an eye-catcher for the general public and probably wouldn't sell very well. Second, leptin is extremely expensive, and given the cost, insurance companies would not cover it even if there were public interest. And last, leptin would only work in conjunction with a diet and exercise program, which further makes the medication less marketable to today's "quick fix" society, which wants to take a few pills and watch the fat melt away. So we can see why supplemental leptin isn't going to be the answer to our problems.

How about the commonly practiced method of dropping calories lower and lower until the scale starts moving again? Well, as you now know, that's probably the worst possible thing anyone could do if continued fat loss is the goal. Further reducing calories will only cause leptin to crash harder, making the metabolic mess these individuals are trying to get out of even worse. Sure, by repeatedly reducing caloric intake over the course of a diet you will eventually lose weight, but much of that weight will end up being muscle (and for those who think training with weights will keep you from losing muscle independent of caloric intake, believe me, the last thing your body is concerned with at such low calorie levels is repairing muscle tissue to maintain muscle mass). The lower you drop calories, the more the body begins to fuel itself on muscle tissue. Why? Because muscle mass is calorically expensive to maintain. That's a good thing under normal circumstances, as muscle promotes a higher resting metabolic rate, but when leptin levels crash, the body is trying to *decrease* energy expenditure, so it begins to feed on muscle mass. A lower degree of muscle mass equals a lower metabolic rate, which is exactly what the body wants in this situation.

This decrease in muscle mass in addition to all the other hormonal and metabolic adaptations is why the percentage of people who are able to keep lost weight off for any substantial amount of time is in the single digits. Prolonged dieting leaves your metabolism so tremendously screwed up that you'd have to continue to diet at extremely low calorie levels for the rest of your life to prevent the weight from piling back on. There has to be a better way to diet, an actual solution—and there is. That way is called Cheat to Lose.

You Want Me to Do *What*?

We know that under normal circumstances leptin is plentiful and the brain senses that everything is A-OK. Metabolic rate is high, hormones are stabilized, and all in all it's a very conducive environment for fat burning. Unfortunately, as we also now know, this fat-burning environment quickly fades as soon as we begin to restrict calories and actually try to strip some fat away. Though our bodies have a pretty good reason for their reaction, it's pretty ironic that they're primed for fat loss at every other time except for when we are trying to lose fat. Wouldn't it be great if we could diet while still maintaining that fat-burning milieu? It would seemingly solve all our problems. To do this, though, we'd have to be able to keep leptin levels normalized in the face of calorie restriction. Well, I have good news for you—there is a way. And the even better news is that you're going to absolutely *love* the solution.

Recall that there is a direct, linear relationship between leptin levels and the amount of food you are eating. A decrease in energy intake yields a decrease in leptin levels, fat loss is decelerated, and all those nasty physiological side effects mentioned earlier begin to set in. But since the relationship is linear, the opposite is also true: an increase in caloric intake will result in an increase in leptin levels. And while leptin levels drop around 50 percent after one week of dieting, it only takes one *day* of overfeeding or "cheating" to bring levels back up to baseline. So the solution to our dilemma and the very premise of this diet is: *cheat!* That's right, on the Cheat to Lose Diet, you will be committing the dietary cardinal sin of throwing the rules out the window and eating the foods you crave on a weekly basis. And for those of you concerned that a day of overfeeding will negate recent progress, have no worries—leptin levels rise faster than lost fat is able to come back on. Moreover, only a few days after the cheat, when the initial water bloat from the caloric surplus has faded, you will find that weight and body fat have measurably decreased.

It all makes perfect physiological and psychological sense. By periodically cheating on your diet, you circumvent the negative physiological side effects of calorie restriction. Each week you start fresh with baseline levels of leptin and a hormonal environment primed for burning fat, not muscle. The metabolic crash that occurs with prolonged dieting is no longer an issue, so keeping lost weight lost as you enter the maintenance phase of the diet won't be a problem.

And forget about psychological feelings like guilt and failure. You don't feel guilty when you cheat, you feel good—because you know that when you do, you're helping to accelerate your progress. Anxiety? Not here; when cravings arise, there is comfort in knowing that you will be able to enjoy that very food when your next cheat rolls around in only a few short days. Feelings of discouragement and decreased motivation? No again; when progress is occurring week in and week out, there's no reason to become discouraged. And many have reported that the psychological vent cheating provides causes them to return to their diets the next day with renewed drive and dedication.

Cheating serves as both a physiological boost and a psychological vent. What's more, from a psychological point of view, cheating allows us to avoid many of the emotional issues that result from a lack of progress (frustration, discouragement, depression, etc.). With Cheat to Lose, cheating is not just something that is "allowed"—it's a vital part of the program's success. Finally, a diet that works with your body, not against it!

References

Ahima RS et al. Role of leptin in the neuroendocrine response to fasting. Nature. 1996 Jul 18;382(6588):250–2.

Ahima RS et al. Leptin regulation of neuroendocrine systems. Front Neuroendocrinology 2000 Jul;21(3):263–307.

Ahima RS, Flier JS. Leptin. Annu Rev Physiol. 2000;62:413–37. Review.

Arhen B et al. Regulation of circulating leptin in humans. Endocrine. 1997 Aug;7(1):1–8. Review.

Blum WF. Leptin: the voice of the adipose tissue. Horm Res. 1997;48 (Suppl 4):2–8. Review.

Boden G et al. Effect of fasting on serum leptin in normal human subjects. J Clin Endocrinol Metab. 1996 Sep;81(9):3419–23.

Bowles L, Kopelman P. Leptin: of mice and men? J Clin Pathol. 2001 Jan; 54(1):1–3

Carantoni M et al. Can changes in plasma insulin concentration explain the variability in leptin response to weight loss in obese women with normal glucose tolerance? J Clin Endocrinol Metab. 1999 Mar;84(3):869–72.

Dirlewanger M et al. Effects of short-term carbohydrate or fat overfeeding on energy expenditure and plasma leptin concentrations in healthy female subjects. Int J Obes Relat Metab Disord. 2000 Nov;24(11):1413–8.

Doucet E et al. Changes in energy expenditure and substrate oxidation resulting from weight loss in obese men and women: is there an important contribution of leptin? J Clin Endocrinol Metab. 2000 Apr;85(4):1550–6.

Douyon L, Schteingart DE. Effect of obesity and starvation on thyroid hormone, growth hormone, and cortisol secretion. Endocrinol Metab Clin North Am. 2002 Mar;31(1):173–89.

Dubuc GR, Havel PJ et al. Changes of serum leptin and endocrine and metabolic parameters after 7 days of energy restriction in men and women. Metabolism. 1998 Apr;47(4):429–34.

Girard J. Is leptin the link between obesity and insulin resistance? Diabetes Metab. 1997 Sep;23 (Suppl 3):16–24. Review.

Haluzik M et al. The influence of short-term fasting on serum leptin levels, and selected hormonal and metabolic parameters in morbidly obese and lean females. Endocr Res. 2001 Feb-May;27(1–2):251–60.

Hamann A, Matthaei S. Regulation of energy balance by leptin. Exp Clin Endocrinol Diabetes. 1996;104(4):293–300. Review.

Havel PJ et al. High-fat meals reduce 24–h circulating leptin concentrations in women. Diabetes. 1999 Feb;48(2):334–41.

Havel PJ et al. Relationship of plasma leptin to plasma insulin and adiposity in normal weight and overweight women: effects of dietary fat content and sustained weight loss. J Clin Endocrinol Metab. 1996 Dec;81(12):4406–13.

Havel PJ. Role of adipose tissue in body-weight regulation: mechanisms regulating leptin production and energy balance. Proc Nutr Soc. 2000 Aug;59(3): 359–71. Review.

Hwa JJ et al. Intracerebroventricular injection of leptin increases thermogenesis and mobilizes fat metabolism in ob/ob mice. Horm Metab Res. 1996 Dec;28(12):659–63.

Jenkins AB et al. Carbohydrate intake and short-term regulation of leptin in humans. Diabetologia. 1997 Mar;40(3):348–51.

Keim NL, Stern JS, Havel PJ. Relation between circulating leptin concentrations and appetite during a prolonged, moderate energy deficit in women. Am J Clin Nutr. 1998 Oct;68(4):794–801.

Kennedy A et al. The metabolic significance of leptin in humans: gender-based differences in relationship to adiposity, insulin sensitivity, and energy expenditure. J Clin Endocrinol Metab. 1997 Apr;82(4):1293–300.

Klein S et al. Leptin production during early starvation in lean and obese women. Am J Physiol Endocrinol Metab. 2000 Feb;278(2):E280–4.

Kolaczynski JW. Response of leptin to short-term and prolonged overfeeding in humans. J Clin Endocrinol Metab. 1996 Nov;81(11):4162–5.

Kolaczynski JW. Responses of leptin to short-term fasting and refeeding in humans: a link with ketogenesis but not ketones themselves. Diabetes. 1996 Nov;45(11):1511–5.

Levin BE, Routh VH. Role of the brain in energy balance and obesity. Am J Physiol. 1996 Sep;271(3 Pt 2):R491–500. Review.

Maffei M, Halaas J et al. Leptin levels in human and rodent: measurement of plasma leptin and ob RNA in obese and weight-reduced subjects. Nat Med. 1995 Nov;1(11):1155–61.

Mars M et al. Fasting leptin and appetite responses induced by a 4-day 65%-energy-restricted diet. Int J Obes (Lond). 2006 Jan;30(1):122–8.

Mars M et al. Leptin and insulin responses to a four-day energy-deficient diet in men with different weight history. Int J Obes Relat Metab Disord. 2003 May;27(5):574–81.

Martinez JA, Fruhbek G. Regulation of energy balance and adiposity: a model with new approaches. Rev Esp Fisiol. 1996 Dec;52(4):255–8. Review.

McGarry JD. Appetite control: Does leptin lighten the problem of obesity? Curr Biol. 1995 Dec 1;5(12):1342–4. Review.

Meinders AE et al. Leptin. Neth J Med. 1996 Dec;49(6):247–52. Review.

Miyawaki T et al. Clinical implications of leptin and its potential humoral regulators in long-term low-calorie diet therapy for obese humans. Eur J Clin Nutr. 2002 Jul;56(7):593–600.

National Centre for Eating Disorders. Psychology of Dieting. 1999.

Nedvidkova J. Leptin. Cesk Fysiol. 1997 Dec;46(4):182–8. Review.

Nicklas BJ et al. Gender differences in the response of plasma leptin concentrations to weight loss in obese older individuals. Obes Res. 1997 Jan;5(1):62–8.

Okazaki T et al. Effects of mild aerobic exercise and a mild hypocaloric diet on plasma leptin in sedentary women. Clin Exp Pharmacol Physiol. 1999 May-Jun;26(5–6):415–20.

Palesty JA. The Goldilocks paradigm of starvation and refeeding. Nutr Clin Pract. 2006 Apr;21(2):147–54. Review.

Pratley RE et al. Plasma leptin responses to fasting in Pima Indians. Am J Physiol. 1997 Sep;273(3 Pt 1):E644–9.

Racette SB, Kohrt WM et al. Response of serum leptin concentrations to 7 d of energy restriction in centrally obese African Americans with impaired or diabetic glucose tolerance. Am J Clin Nutr. 1997 Jul;66(1):33–7.

Reseland JE et al. Effect of long-term changes in diet and exercise on plasma leptin concentrations. Am J Clin Nutr. 2001 Feb;73(2):240–5.

Rohner-Jeanrenaud E, Jeanrenaud B. Central nervous system and body weight regulation. Ann Endocrinol (Paris). 1997;58(2):137–42. Review.

Romon M et al. Leptin response to carbohydrate or fat meal and association with subsequent satiety and energy intake. Am J Physiol. 1999 Nov;277(5 Pt 1): E855–61.

Rosenbaum M et al. Low-dose leptin administration reverses effects of sustained weight-reduction on energy expenditure and circulating concentrations of thyroid hormones. J Clin Endocrinol Metab. 2002; 87:2391–2394.

Rowland NE, Morien A, Li BH. The physiology and brain mechanisms of feeding. Nutrition. 1996 Sep;12(9):626–39. Review.

Salidin R et al. Transient increase in obese gene expression after food intake or insulin administration. Nature. 1995 Oct 12;377(6549):527–9.

Schwartz MW, Seeley RJ. The new biology of body weight regulation. J Am Diet Assoc. 1997 Jan;97(1):54–8; quiz 59–60. Review.

Smith SR. The endocrinology of obesity. Endocrinol Metab Clin North Am. 1996 Dec;25(4):921–42. Review.

Spitzweg C, Joba W, Heufelder AE. Leptin—new knowledge on the pathogenesis of obesity. Med Klin (Munich). 1998 Aug 15;93(8):478–85. Review.

Tuominen et al. Leptin and thermogenesis in humans. Acta Physiol Scand. 1997 May;160(1):83–7.

van Aggel-Leijssen DP et al. Regulation of average 24h human plasma leptin level; the influence of exercise and physiological changes in energy balance. Int J Obes Relat Metab Disord. 1999 Feb;23(2):151–8.

van Dijk G. The role of leptin in regulation of energy balance and adiposity. J Neuroendocrinol. 2001 Oct;13(10):913–21.

Weigle DS et al. Effect of fasting, refeeding, and dietary fat restriction on plasma leptin levels. J Clin Endocrinol Metab. 1997 Feb;82(2):561–5.

Wing RR et al. Relationship between weight loss maintenance and changes in serum leptin levels. Horm Metab Res. 1996 Dec;28(12):698–703.

Wolf G. Leptin: the weight-reducing plasma protein encoded by the obese gene. Nutr Rev. 1996 Mar;54(3):91–3. Review.

Zimmet P. Serum leptin concentration, obesity, and insulin resistance in Western Samoans: cross sectional study. BMJ. 1996 Oct 19;313(7063):965–9.

3

Choosing the Right Fats and Carbs

This is the leanest I've ever been! Thanks to the Cheat to Lose Diet, I've reached my goal of losing 15 pounds of fat, and each week have had to move down another hole on my belt. And it wasn't even that hard! I've tried other diets, like the low-carb approach, but they just weren't realistic for the long term—there was nothing to look forward to, only more dieting. With Cheat to Lose, I had plenty of carbs and tasty meals during the week to keep me going and then a Cheat Day each week when I was able to eat literally anything and as much as I wanted. This is something I can see myself doing for the rest of my life.

Paul N.

Canberra, Australia

In 2003, I went from just over 300 pounds to just under 200 via very-low-carb dieting, but was struggling to lose any additional weight. As a matter of fact, when I tried to reintroduce carbs to my daily diet, my weight shot back up 30 pounds! For months I struggled to find a balance between consuming some sort of "normal" diet and achieving the weight loss I was hoping for, but feared I had done too much damage to my metabolism over the past year. Months went by without my achieving any real results, and then I began the Cheat to Lose Diet under Joel's supervision. Not only did this diet help to restore my "dead" metabolism, but it helped me to effortlessly lose just over 25 unwanted inches from my body!

Pamela J.
Sealy, Texas

As a personal trainer, I have been on a diet most of my adult life. That said, dieting has always left me feeling deprived, never satisfied. After all, diets are generally restrictive in nature, all about the foods you can't eat. In contrast, the Cheat to Lose Diet is about what you can eat, and it even goes a step beyond to teach you how you can make literally any and every type of food part of your life. In eight weeks, CTL has helped me achieve my leanest conditioning, assisting me in dropping an additional 9 inches from my frame. And the best part—I was able to drop my regular diet and am now enjoying eating a wide variety of foods on a weekly basis. I'm no longer feeling deprived, and that's a great feeling.

Kori B., certified personal trainer
Waukesha, Wisconsin

Having been overweight literally my entire life, I had tried just about every weight-loss method, from low-carb to low-fat. Nothing worked—that is, until I took a chance on the Cheat to Lose Diet. Who would have thought that regularly "cheating" on my diet would yield these kinds of results? Because of Cheat to Lose, I'm currently at the lowest level of body fat I've ever been (for the first time in my life, I can see my abs!) and with more confidence and energy than ever before. Everyone has been asking me what I've been doing to lose weight; they can't believe the answer when I tell them what I've been eating every Sunday. Talk about an easy, extremely effective way to achieve your goals—this diet is a godsend!

Stuart K., Ph.D.
London, England

Before we get into the specifics of the diet, I want to talk about two things that the Cheat to Lose Diet is *not:* low-fat or low-carb. While the average American's intake of unhealthy fats and highly refined carbohydrates is much too high, recommending extreme limitation of an entire macronutrient is unnecessary and ends up doing more harm than good. Simply put, anytime you eliminate 95 percent of what you're "allowed" to eat, chances are your diet is not optimal, and is probably unhealthy. A much better solution would be to teach individuals how to choose the right *types* of fats and carbs—and that's exactly what I'm going to teach *you* over the course of this next chapter.

The Low-Fat Diet

Prior to our discussion of "good" and "bad" fats and carbs, I'd like to briefly delve into the shortcomings of the low-fat and low-carb approaches to dieting, respectively. Diets low in fat haven't done very much at all to support America's efforts toward permanent weight loss and better health. Despite the fact that our grocery store shelves have been overflowing with low-fat and no-fat food-stuffs for the past two decades, obesity levels have continued to climb higher and higher—not exactly the result low-fat advocates were hoping for. The recommendation to lower fat intake was shortsighted and perpetuated a host of negative side effects (from both health and fat-loss standpoints) that continue to plague followers of the approach today.

Let's take a look at the first aim of low-fat diets: to decrease the risk of developing the number one and number two killers in the United States—cardiovascular disease and cancer. When research linking the consumption of certain types of fats to these diseases emerged, health professionals huddled together to design a plan to get Americans to reduce their intake of those types of fat. Their response was to recommend lowering fat intake across the board in order to keep things simple. Unfortunately, this oversimplification also caused individuals to reduce their consumption of other types of fat—fat possessing many health benefits, including anti-cancer and anti-heart-disease properties. Moreover, recent, long-term, comprehensive research (the Women's Health Initiative Trial, which studied 40,000 women over eight years) found that low-fat diets did not significantly reduce the occurrence of cardiovascular disease and cancer.

And then there is reason number two: to promote fat loss and reap the health benefits associated with reduced levels of body fat. Because fat is the most calorically dense macronutrient, providing 9 calories per gram (more than twice the calorie load of carbohydrates or protein), it was theorized that reducing fat intake would cause fat loss by removing a large portion of calories from the average diet. Contrary to this line of thinking, as we discussed earlier, calorie reduction by itself fails to yield considerable fat loss due to the body's reaction to such reductions. Even with that aside (and it's a *big* one), a large amount of fat loss is not likely to occur on a very-low-fat diet due to the hormonal crash associated with such nutritional regimens. Substantial fat intake is necessary to promote optimal levels of anabolic hormones (responsible for maintaining and building muscle mass, among other things), and levels of these hormones are anything but optimal on a low-fat diet. Low anabolic hormone levels + reduced calories = muscle loss. Muscle loss = a decrease in metabolic rate = further difficulty losing fat and keeping it off.

In addition, there is the issue of replacement. Not only are low-fat dieters missing out on the benefits of healthy fats, but in their place they're consuming large quantities of worthless, health-demoting, insulin-spiking, fat-storage-promoting carbohydrates. Processed reduced-fat snack crackers and potato chips; sugar-laden low-fat or fat-free cereals, cookies, ice cream, and candy; and white bread, bagels, and pretzels are just a few of the extremely refined carb sources these individuals have been led to believe are healthy food choices. Couple this consumption with a hormonal environment that makes us prone to fat gain and we can begin to see why low-fat diets have been highly unsuccessful at treating obesity.

Still, there are other problems. Fat is believed to be the most satiating of the three macronutrients, and continually limiting its consumption leaves dieters feeling deprived. Any nutritional regimen that leaves its followers with constant feelings of hunger, regardless of its proposed efficacy, is not a very practical approach to weight loss. And going back to the hormonal crash resulting from a low fat intake, there are other side effects, including lethargy, low sex drive, and impaired sexual function.

To summarize, low-fat diets:

- Cause dieters to miss out on the many benefits of healthy fats
- Often have dieters replacing calories from fat with highly refined carb sources
- Often leave dieters feeling unsatisfied and hungry
- Cause crashing hormone levels that exacerbate common side effects of a reduced calorie intake such as muscle loss, lethargy, and sexual side effects

Clearly, limiting all dietary fat is not the way to go about reducing the intake of "bad" fats. As mentioned earlier, the more logical solution is to keep a tight rein on those fats whose consumption poses a health risk while continuing to enjoy those with health benefits.

The Low-Carb Diet

Low-carb advocates (in conjunction with the media) have done a magnificent job of brainwashing the American public into believing that all carbohydrates are evil, when in fact the resolution to the carbohydrate conundrum is again not to avoid the macronutrient altogether, but rather to choose the *right types* of carbohydrates to consume.

The low-carb diet was founded on the theory that limiting the intake of the body's primary source of energy, carbohydrates, would force the body to rely on its secondary source, fat, for fuel and thus would promote greater fat loss than more conventional dieting methods. While it sounds logical, it doesn't quite work out that way, and when we think things through a little more thoroughly, we see why this is the case. Yes, low-carb diets limit energy intake from carbohydrates, but to compensate for the decrease in carbs, fat intake is increased. Therefore low-carb dieters eat more fat on a daily basis, and the body begins to burn the additional fat consumed instead of the stored body fat these individuals are trying to do away with. So yes, limiting carbs will cause the body to rely on fat for fuel, but by replacing those carbs with fat, it's simply taking one step forward and one step back.

But what about the tremendous weight loss reported by low-carb dieters, especially after the first month of dieting? Down 18 pounds in four weeks! Down 12 pounds in two and a half weeks! How could a diet producing such dramatic results be deemed ineffective? Well, here's where we need to start differentiating between weight loss and fat loss. *Weight loss* is a blanket term, one that can apply to weight reduction resulting from the loss of a variety of substances in the body. One of these substances is glycogen—unscientifically put, stored carbohydrate within the body. Carbohydrate is stored both in the liver and in muscle tissue as a source of immediate energy for the body to tap when in need. In the absence of carbohydrate ingestion (or when ingestion is limited), glycogen stores can become depleted in as little as a few days. Additionally, much of the weight lost during the first few weeks of low-carb dieting is water weight. Anytime one embarks on a diet, some water loss is expected as a result of the reduced calorie intake, but restricting carbohydrate intake in conjunction with calories leads to a much more pronounced loss in water mass. Next, there is an issue that was touched on briefly in the last chapter—muscle loss. Many low-carb dieters make the mistake of reducing their caloric intake well below their needs, perpetuating losses in muscle mass. And lastly, we have the obvious—fat loss. Fat is generally what low-carb dieters believe they are losing when the number on the scale begins to fall; however, as we are now learning, losses in glycogen, water, and muscle mass play a major role in that figure taking a dive, especially during the initial stages of the diet.

Below is a sample weight-loss breakdown for someone claiming a 12-pound loss during the first two and a half weeks of his or her low-carb diet:

Water loss: 8 pounds
Glycogen loss:
   1 pound
Muscle loss:
   1.5 pounds
Fat loss: 1.5 pounds

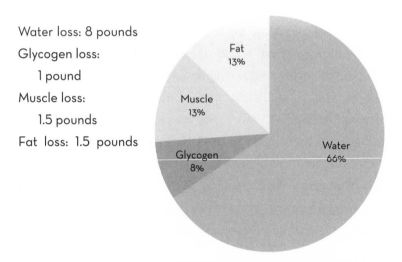

As you can see, a very small percentage of the weight lost in the above example is from fat, giving the individual in question a false sense of accomplishment. And that's what low-carb diets do—entice the uninformed with initial results that are seemingly unheard of, only to let these same individuals down in the weeks and months to come as weight loss begins to slow considerably.

Low-carb dieting presents a much bigger problem than just giving individuals a false sense of results, and that problem is the negative impact it has on leptin. This is a result of another hormone, insulin, being chronically low during low-carb dieting. Insulin is a "storage" hormone released from the pancreas in response to carbohydrate ingestion. After ingestion, carbohydrate is broken down into its simplest form (sugar) and is then released into the bloodstream. Insulin's function is to remove the sugar from the bloodstream and deliver it to the proper storage site (either muscle or fat). Now, while chronically *high* levels of insulin are certainly undesirable from a fat storage and health risk standpoint, extremely *low* levels of insulin day in and day out are just as undesirable for the dieter, and here's why: research has shown leptin to be positively correlated with insulin. In other words, insulin helps to offset that red flag message being sent to the brain while dieting (this is a major reason why periodic cheating works so well). Because there is very little carbohydrate being consumed on a low-carb diet, insulin is chronically low (the key word is *chronically*). And because insulin is chronically low, leptin levels suffer. Chronic low-carb intake = chronic low insulin levels = suffering leptin levels.

The last and perhaps biggest strike against the low-carb diet is the approach's extreme impracticality. To adhere to such a regimen, followers must fight—on a daily basis—not only the general cravings associated with calorie restriction, but also intense carbohydrate cravings for foods that they *should be allowed to eat*. To say that dieters are not permitted to enjoy foods such as pasta, potatoes, whole grains, and many fruits and vegetables is both impractical and unnecessary. Practicality comes down to sacrifice (investment) versus results (return), and unfortunately the low-carb diet is unable to produce the results necessary to counterbalance the immense sacrifice required.

To recap, low-carb diets:

- Give dieters a false sense of progress through weight loss, not fat loss
- Negatively impact leptin, exacerbating the metabolic adaptations that occur while dieting
- Fail to produce the results necessary to make such an extreme diet worthwhile

Now that we've cleared up the false notion that fats and carbs as a whole are "bad," let's take a look at the types of each nutrient you should be regularly consuming and those you should be wary of.

Choosing the Right Fats

The problems with dietary fat and cholesterol arise when we consume fats and cholesterol that have been damaged or oxidized by heat, oxygen, and light. Oxidized fats and cholesterol contain high amounts of dangerous free radicals that contribute to the buildup of plaque in arteries and damage to the arterial wall, as well as the development of certain cancers. Up until a few generations ago, denatured fats and cholesterol were few and far between (and interestingly enough, the incidence of heart disease was low), as the majority of dietary fats consumed prior to the mid-1900s were "natural" and not victims of the extreme processing methods used today. For example, instead of the old method of gently pressing oil from its source, today seeds and the like are crushed and then heated to extreme temperatures to extract their oil. Such extreme

Basic Types of Fat

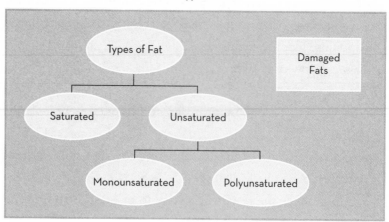

temperatures wreak havoc on the fragile fats of these oils, leaving the final product denatured and full of dangerous free radicals.

Hydrogenation is another common processing method that is detrimental to fats that are exposed to it. In this process, hydrogen is bubbled through naturally occurring unsaturated fats, transforming them into the man-made dietary demon known as transfatty acids or trans fats. Because trans-fatty acids do not occur in nature (with rare exceptions), our bodies are not equipped with mechanisms to deal with them once ingested. Even an extremely small intake of trans fats has been shown to result in negative health consequences; however, consumption among the American public is anything but small. Trans fats are everywhere. They are commonly used as a preservative to increase the shelf life of packaged goods, and are frequently substituted for saturated fats in many products to give consumers the ridiculously false impression that these products are healthier. Consumption of trans fats has been linked to many diseases and health problems including heart disease, cancer, diabetes, immune dysfunction, and dementia. It is important to read all labels very carefully, strictly avoiding any product containing "hydrogenated" or partially hydrogenated oils in its list of ingredients. Other sources of trans fat include foods that have been deep-fried at high temperatures (fried chicken, french fries, etc.).

Omega-6 and Omega-3 Fatty Acids: Too Much and Too Little of a Good Thing

Omega-6 and omega-3 fatty acids are polyunsaturated fats that are considered to be *essential* (meaning the body is unable to make them and they can only be obtained by dietary means). Omega-3 fatty acids possess a myriad of health benefits but, as a result of modern processing and agriculture, are scarce in the American food supply. They are abundant in oils from cold-water fish, however, and can also be found in more moderate amounts in flaxseeds and flaxseed products. Omega-3s are extremely delicate and prone to rancidity; therefore, unless encapsulated, they should be refrigerated and stored in containers where their exposure to light is minimal. To name just a few of the health benefits these "wonder" fats possess, they have been shown to decrease the risk for developing heart disease and cancer, decrease blood pressure, improve liver and kidney function, reduce joint pain, improve vision, improve diabetic conditions, decrease the frequency and the intensity of migraine headaches, increase circulating levels of leptin, reduce stress, and increase metabolic rate.

However, the average American intake of omega-6 fatty acids greatly exceeds what is necessary, while the intake of omega-3s leaves much to be desired. Just about every source of fat we can consume contains at least some omega-6 fatty acids (animal products, vegetable oils, nuts, etc.), but very few sources contain substantial amounts of omega-3s, leaving the typical American diet with an omega-6-to-omega-3 ratio of 10:1 or even 20:1, when the ideal is somewhere in the 3:1 to 1:1 range.

Research has shown that excessive consumption of omega-6s can have adverse health effects (mostly as a result of the pro-inflammatory properties of these fatty acids), so it's best not to overindulge. Instead, don't plan on eating them and you'll likely obtain all that you need.

Again, you'll get plenty of polyunsaturated fats, especially the omega-6 variety, through regular dietary consumption, but you may have to take a supplemental approach to ensure that you are getting enough omega-3s, especially if you are not regularly consuming fish as a protein source.

Monounsaturated Fat

Monounsaturated fats are relatively stable, making them a good choice for cooking at moderate temperatures. They have been shown to boost immune function, support healthy hormone levels, and decrease the risk for developing cancer and heart disease. Additionally, olive oil—a great source of monounsaturated fat—is rich in antioxidants, particularly vitamin E, which further fight disease and aging by attacking dangerous free radicals. Just be sure to choose extra-virgin olive oil, which is extracted through a gentler process than other commercial olive oils, leaving the fats and antioxidants it contains undamaged. Other good sources of monounsaturates include canola oil, almonds and almond butter, avocados, hazelnuts, pecans, and Brazil nuts.

Saturated Fat and Animal Fat

Often we are advised to avoid red meat and other animal products because of their saturated fat content. In fact, the terms *saturated fat* and *animal fat* are used almost interchangeably by the media and many health professionals today. While avoiding an excessive intake of saturated fats is a good idea in general, most anti-beef advocates fail to realize that more than half of the fat in red meat is unsaturated. Furthermore, the most common saturate found in beef and dairy products is stearic acid, consumption of which has been shown to decrease plasma and liver cholesterol by reducing intestinal cholesterol absorption. Also, stearic acid intake helps to prevent arterial clotting and the formation of fatty deposits within the arteries, so don't let the hype deter you from sitting down every so often to enjoy a tender, flavorful steak.

A Carb Is a Carb Is a—*I Don't Think So!*

So far in this chapter we've discussed both low-fat and low-carb diets, their shortcomings, and the various benefits of including both macronutrients in the diet. You now should also have a better idea of which fats are healthy to consume and which you should strive to avoid. The only thing left to do now is talk about how to choose the *right* carbs.

As was the case with fats, not all carbohydrates are created equal, and while lumping all carbs together as "bad" isn't very astute, treating them all as "good" would also be a rather big mistake. The issue with carbohydrates is how fast a particular carb source is broken down to its simplest form, glucose (a type of sugar), and released into the bloodstream. For example, highly refined carbohydrates such as white bread and simple sugars are digested quickly and enter the blood at a relatively rapid rate, while fiber-rich, unrefined sources tend to be digested more slowly and yield a steady, controlled release of glucose. Typically, a spike in blood glucose yields a spike in the hormone insulin (recall that insulin is a storage hormone released from the pancreas whose function is to clear glucose from the bloodstream), while a steady release of glucose into the bloodstream yields a steady, controlled release of insulin (though there are exceptions, which we will discuss shortly). As mentioned earlier, chronically high levels of insulin caused by regularly consuming highly refined carbs and simple sugars can be detrimental both to your fat-burning efforts and to your overall health. Spikes in insulin lead to more fat storage and less fat burning. Also, regular consumption of insulin-spiking foods can lower your sensitivity to insulin, a condition that can eventually result in type II diabetes. So "good" carbs would be those that are digested slowly and have a low insulin response, and "bad" carbs are those that spike blood sugar and cause the pancreas to pour out massive amounts of insulin.

But how do you know what effect a certain carb source has on blood sugar and insulin? How can you tell one carb from another? Certainly a bit of common sense comes into play here, as one could probably tell that the carbs found in broccoli are a lot healthier and have much less impact on blood sugar and insulin than do the carbs found in potato chips or some other kind of junk food. Some carb sources and their glycemic effects aren't as clear-cut, though, bringing about the need for some sort of classification system. Over the years, a few have been used; let's take a look.

Simple versus Complex

The simple-versus-complex classification scheme was the first used to distinguish between "good" and "bad" carbs and did so by chemical structure. A carbohydrate was considered "simple" if it had a relatively simple chemical makeup, that is, somewhere between one and nine carbohydrate molecules linked together. If the carbohydrate was made up of ten or more molecules, it was labeled as "complex." The idea was that if a carb source was composed of many molecules linked together, it should take longer to digest and would be released slowly into the bloodstream, yielding a controlled, moderate insulin response. Similarly, if a carb source had a simple makeup of less than ten molecules, then it should be digested rapidly, causing the pancreas to produce a large amount of insulin to clear the blood of the abundance of sugar. Unfortunately, things once again didn't quite work out as theorized. When put to the test, researchers discovered that some chemically complex carb sources, such as white potatoes and other starches, are digested quickly, spiking blood sugar and insulin, while some simple carb sources, such as fructose (one of the sugars found in fruit) and certain legumes, are digested slowly and have a more subtle impact on blood sugar and insulin. These findings made it clear that the chemical structure of a particular carb source wasn't a good indicator of how fast that source gives rise to blood sugar, and paved the way for the development of something much more useful—the glycemic index.

Glycemic Index

The glycemic index (GI) is a system in which foods are ranked according to how fast they cause blood sugar to rise. Instead of relying on theory to hypothesize this speed, the glycemic index is derived from data that measure the speed directly. With the GI system, each food is assigned a numerical value that is representative of the food's effect on blood sugar relative to the standard, glucose (there is also a scale in which white bread is the standard; however, it is not as common nor as useful since there are numerous foods that are digested more rapidly than white bread and so end up having higher values than the standard). Because glucose is the simplest sugar and is the compound all carbs are converted to before being released into the bloodstream, it makes for a pretty good standard. On the GI scale, glucose is assigned the value of 100, and as stated previously, all other values are relative to this figure. For example, oat bran has a GI of 50, meaning that oat bran is digested and its sugars released into the bloodstream at half the rate of glucose. To give more meaning to these numbers, a GI of 55 or less is considered low, GIs between 55 and 70 are labeled as moderate, and anything 70 or above constitutes a high GI. As we have mentioned several times in this chapter, we want to choose foods that elicit a steady, controlled blood sugar response, so low-to-moderate-GI foods are the carbs of choice in most circumstances. (That said, certain higher-GI carbs are acceptable when strategically incorporated at specific times; more on this later.) Still, although more advanced and accurate than the simple-versus-complex system, the glycemic index presents a few problems that can be improved upon, as we'll discuss next.

Glycemic Load

The major problem with the glycemic index is that the value assigned to each food is based on a 50-gram sample of carbohydrate, when in most real-world situations it is unlikely that you would eat exactly 50 grams of carbohydrate from a particular food (one could eat much less or much more). Obviously, 50 grams of carbohydrate is going to have a greater impact on blood sugar than, say, 20 grams, and 75 grams more so than 50 grams—the blood sugar response is dependent on the amount of carbohydrate ingested. This sometimes causes the glycemic index to assign a high value to certain foods when in fact it is unlikely that one would consume anywhere near 50 grams of carbohydrate from that food in a single sitting. For example, the GI of cantaloupe is 70, making it a high-GI food (a food that we'd want to avoid in most cases given that number); however, the typical serving size of cantaloupe (1 cup of cubes) contains 13 grams of carbohydrate, not 50. When serving size is considered, cantaloupe's effect on blood sugar becomes much less a concern.

Taking the above into consideration, a new ranking system was developed—glycemic load (GL). Glycemic load is similar to the glycemic index in that it measures the effect of a particular carbohydrate on blood sugar; however, it is standardized to typical serving sizes and not an absolute number of grams. On the glycemic load scale, a GL of 10 or less is considered low, between 10 and 20 is medium, and values of 20 and over are high. (See www.glycemicindex.com.)

Insulin Index

While glycemic load does a pretty good job of predicting insulin response based on how fast a particular carb source gives rise to blood sugar, the insulin index (II) takes things one step further by measuring the insulin response of foods directly. In most cases, there is a direct relationship between a food's GL and its II; however, there are a few instances in which the relationship is far from linear. How can this be? Well, it seems that there is more to a food's insulin response than simply how fast that food is digested and assimilated into the bloodstream. Now, before you go throwing the GL scale out the window, please note that there are only a few exceptions to the glycemic load/insulin index parallel. Those exceptions are mainly milk products and foods containing both highly processed carbs and fats (i.e., bakery products, potato chips, pizza, ice cream—pretty much all those things that are common-sense foods to avoid while dieting except on Cheat Days).

Milk products score very low on the glycemic load scale but very high with respect to insulin response. That said, fat-free milk and other dairy products can be beneficial to us as dieters. As stated earlier, insulin has a positive effect on leptin; unfortunately, *regularly* consuming high-calorie, very high-glycemic-index foods in order to generate a significant insulin response isn't going to help our fat-loss efforts very much (we'll save those foods for Cheat Days). However, with dairy products we have foods that can be used throughout the week to give insulin and leptin a bump without a great deal of damage occurring. With these foods, we get the insulin response (which, because of its effect on leptin, helps to offset that red flag message we spoke of previously) without a load of calories and fat storage. Still, dairy products should be used in moderation, as chronically high insulin is detrimental to fat burning and overall health regardless of the calorie content of the food generating the response.

Adding fat to a refined carb source (as is done with most junk foods) tends to slow digestion and therefore the glycemic response; however, it actually *increases* the insulin response associated with that particular food/meal. This helps explain why such foods typically work very well for the planned cheating done on the Cheat to Lose Diet.

Chapter Cheat Sheet

- Effective dieting is about choosing the right fats and carbs, not eliminating them.
- Value cold-water fish oils for their many health benefits.
- Consume modest amounts of olive oil and other monounsaturates.
- Enjoy beef and most other animal fat in addition to and in balance with the above.
- Do not strive to consume additional omega-6 fatty acids, particularly highly concentrated sources such as vegetable oils and vegetable oil spreads.
- Avoid partially hydrogenated oils, deep-fried meats, and other sources of damaged fats.
- Strive to consume foods in the low and moderate categories of the glycemic index and glycemic load scales to keep blood sugar and insulin under control. (Consuming certain higher-GI/GL carbs is acceptable and beneficial when done properly, which will be discussed extensively in the specifics of the diet.)
- The bulk of carbs in your diet should be from fibrous, unrefined sources such as oatmeal, oat bran, lentils, beans, 100 percent

whole-wheat bread, pastas, new potatoes, yams, greens, most other vegetables, and fruit. (A comprehensive list of acceptable carb sources is given in chapter 6.)

- Use fat-free milk and other dairy products in moderation throughout the week to give insulin and subsequently leptin a bump without a great deal of caloric damage.

Now that our discussion of carbs and fats has come to a close, let's jump into some specifics of how you follow the Cheat to Lose Diet.

References

Ahrens E et al. The influence of dietary fats on serum lipid levels in man. Lancet. 1957;1:943–953.

Albertazzi P, Coupland K. Polyunsaturated fatty acids. Is there a role in post-menopausal osteoporosis prevention? Maturitas. 2002 May 20;42(1):13–22.

Aro A et al. Stearic acid, trans fatty acids, and dairy fat: effects on serum and lipoprotein lipids, apolipoproteins, lipoprotein (a), and lipid transfer proteins in healthy subjects. Am J Clin Nutr. 1997;65:1419.

ASCN/AIN Task Force on Trans Fatty Acids: Position paper on trans fatty acids. Am J Clin Nutr. 1996;63:663.

Atkins and other low-carbohydrate diets: hoax or an effective tool for weight loss? Lancet. 2004 Sep 4–10;364(9437):897–9. Review.

Augustsson K, Michaud DS, Rimm EB, Leitzmann MF, Stampfer MJ, Willett WC, Giovannucci E. A prospective study of intake of fish and marine fatty acids and prostate cancer. Cancer Epidemiol Biomarkers Prev. 2003 Jan;12(1):64–7.

Barbosa DS, Cecchini R, El Kadri MZ, Rodriguez MA, Burini RC, Dichi I. Decreased oxidative stress in patients with ulcerative colitis supplemented with fish oil omega-3 fatty acids. Nutrition. 2003 Oct;19(10):837–42.

Belluzzi A, Brignola C, Campieri M, Pera A, Boschi S, Miglioli M. Effect of an enteric-coated fish-oil preparation on relapses in Crohn's disease. N Engl J Med. 1996 Jun 13; 334(24):1557–60.

Berardi J. The Real World (of Physique Research), Part 3. Testosterone Magazine. 8 Aug 2003. http://www.t-mag.com/nation_articles/273real.jsp.

Beresford SAA et al. Low-fat dietary pattern and risk of colorectal cancer: The Women's Health Initiative Randomized Controlled Dietary Modification Trial. Journal of the American Medical Association. 2006 Feb 8;295:643–54.

Berglund L et al. HDL-subpopulation patterns in response to reductions in dietary total and saturated fat intakes in healthy subjects. Am J Clin Nutr. 1999 Dec;70(6):992–1000.

Bhatnagar D, Durrington PN. Omega-3 fatty acids: their role in the prevention and treatment of atherosclerosis related risk factors and complications. Int J Clin Pract. 2003 May;57(4):305–14

Burdge GC, Wootton SA. Conversion of alpha-linolenic acid to eicosapentaenoic, docosapentaenoic and docosahexaenoic acids in young women. Br J Nutr. 2002 Oct;88(4):411–20.

Calder PC. n-3 polyunsaturated fatty acids and cytokine production in health and disease. Ann Nutr Metab. 1997;41(4):203–34.

Carantoni M et al. Can changes in plasma insulin concentration explain the variability in leptin response to weight loss in obese women with normal glucose tolerance? J Clin Endocrinol Metab. 1999 Mar;84(3):869–72.

Cellini M, Caramazza N, Mangiafico P, Possati GL, Caramazza R. Fatty acid use in glaucomatous optic neuropathy treatment. Acta Ophthalmol Scand Suppl. 1998;(227):41–2.

Cha MC, Jones PJ. Dietary fat type and energy restriction interactively influence plasma leptin concentration in rats. J Lipid Res. 1998;39(8):1655–60.

Chicco A, D'Alessandro, ME, Karabatas L, Gutman R, Lombardo, YB. Effect of moderate levels of dietary fish oil on insulin secretion and sensitivity, and pancreas insulin content in normal rats. Ann Nutr Metab. 1996;40(2): 61–70.

Cho SH et al. Clinical efficacy and safety of Lyprinol, a patented extract from New Zealand green-lipped mussel (Perna Canaliculus) in patients with osteoarthritis of the hip and knee: a multicenter 2-month clinical trial. Allerg Immunol (Paris). 2003 Jun;35(6):212–6.

Collett ED, Davidson LA, Fan YY, Lupton JR, Chapkin RS. n-6 and n-3 polyunsaturated fatty acids differentially modulate oncogenic Ras activation in colonocytes. Am J Physiol Cell Physiol. 2001 May;280(5):C1066–75.

Collier G, O'Dea K. The effect of coingestion of fat on the glucose, insulin and gastric inhibitory peptide responses to carbohydrate and protein. Am J Clin Nutr. 1983 Jun;37(6):941–4.

Cunnane SC, Ho SY, Dore-Duffy P, Ells KR, Horrobin DF. Essential fatty acid and lipid profiles in plasma and erythrocytes in patients with multiple sclerosis. Am J Clin Nutr. 1989 Oct;50(4):801–6.

Curtis CL et al. Effects of n-3 fatty acids on cartilage metabolism. Proc Nutr Soc. 2002 Aug;61(3):381–9.

Curtis CL et al. Pathologic indicators of degradation and inflammation in human osteoarthritic cartilage are abrogated by exposure to n-3 fatty acids. Arthritis Rheum. 2002 Jun;46(6):1544–53.

Das UN. Beneficial effect of eicosapentaenoic and docosahexaenoic acids in the management of systemic lupus erythematosus and its relationship to the cytokine network. Prostaglandins Leukot Essent Fatty Acids. 1994 Sep;51 (3):207–13.

Davis BC, Kris-Etherton PM. Achieving optimal essential fatty acid status in vegetarians: current knowledge and practical implications. Am J Clin Nutr. 2003 Sep;78(3 Suppl):640S–6.

De Vizia B et al. Effect of an 8–month treatment with omega-3 fatty acids (eicosapentaenoic and docosahexaenoic) in patients with cystic fibrosis. JPEN J Parenter Enteral Nutr. 2003 Jan-Feb;27(1):52–7.

Delarue J, Matzinger O, Binnert C, Schneiter P, Chiolero R, Tappy L. Fish oil prevents the adrenal activation elicited by mental stress in healthy men. Diabetes Metab. 2003 Jun;29(3):289–95.

Dietary fat intake and risk of type 2 diabetes in women. Am J Clin Nutr. 2001 Jun;73(6):1019–26.

DiGiacomo RA, Kremer JM, Shah DM. Fish-oil dietary supplementation in patients with Raynaud's phenomenon: a double-blind, controlled, prospective study. Am J Med. 1989 Feb;86(2):158–64.

Dirlewanger M et al. Effects of short-term carbohydrate or fat overfeeding on energy expenditure and plasma leptin concentrations in healthy female subjects. Int J Obes Relat Metab Disord. 2000 Nov;24(11):1413–8.

Donadio JV. n-3 Fatty acids and their role in nephrologic practice. Curr Opin Nephrol Hypertens. 2001 Sep;10(5):639–42.

Dorgan JF et al. Effects of dietary fat and fiber on plasma and urine androgens and estrogens in men: a controlled feeding study. Am J Clin Nutr. 1996 Dec;64(6):850–5.

Dunstan JA et al. Fish oil supplementation in pregnancy modifies neonatal allergen-specific immune responses and clinical outcomes in infants at high risk of atopy: A randomized, controlled trial. J Allergy Clin Immunol. 2003 Dec;112(6):1178–84.

Durrington PN et al. An omega-3 polyunsaturated fatty acid concentrate administered for one year decreased triglycerides in simvastatin treated patients with coronary heart disease and persisting hypertriglyceridaemia. Heart. 2001 May;85(5):544–8.

Engler MM et al. Effects of docosahexaenoic acid on vascular pathology and reactivity in hypertension. Exp Biol Med (Maywood). 2003 Mar;228(3):299–307.

Ernst E. Complementary and alternative medicine in rheumatology. Baillieres Best Pract Res Clin Rheumatol. 2000 Dec;14(4):731–49.

Fernandez-Real JM, Broch M, Vendrell J, Ricart W. Insulin resistance, inflammation, and serum fatty acid composition. Diabetes Care. 2003 May;26(5): 1362–8.

Gago-Dominguez M, Yuan JM, Sun CL, Lee HP, Yu MC. Opposing effects of dietary n-3 and n-6 fatty acids on mammary carcinogenesis: The Singapore Chinese Health Study. Br J Cancer. 2003 Nov 3;89(9):1686–92.

Gallai V et al. Cytokine secretion and eicosanoid production in the peripheral blood mononuclear cells of MS patients undergoing dietary supplementation with n-3 polyunsaturated fatty acids. J Neuroimmunol. 1995 Feb;56(2):143–53.

Garg A et al. Comparison of a high-carbohydrate diet with a high-monounsaturated-fat diet in patients with non-insulin-dependent diabetes mellitus. N Engl J Med. 1988 Sep 29;319(13):829–34.

Ghafoorunissa. Requirements of dietary fats to meet nutritional needs & prevent the risk of atherosclerosis—an Indian perspective. Indian J Med Res. 1998 Nov;108:191–202. Review.

Glew RH et al. The fatty acid composition of the serum phospholipids of children with sickle cell disease in Nigeria. Prostaglandins Leukot Essent Fatty Acids. 2002 Oct;67(4):217–22.

Grimminger F et al. A double-blind, randomized, placebo-controlled trial of n-3 fatty acid based lipid infusion in acute, extended guttate psoriasis. Rapid improvement of clinical manifestations and changes in neutrophil leukotriene profile. Clin Investig. 1993 Aug;71(8):634–43.

Hamalainen E et al. Diet and serum sex hormones in healthy men. J Steroid Biochem. 1984 Jan;20(1):459–64.

Hamalainen EK et al. Decrease of serum total and free testosterone during a low-fat high-fibre diet. J Steroid Biochem. 1983 Mar;18(3):369–370.

Harel Z, Gascon G, Riggs S, Vaz R, Brown W, Exil G. Supplementation with omega-3 polyunsaturated fatty acids in the management of recurrent migraines in adolescents. J Adolesc Health. 2002 Aug;31(2):154–61.

Harper CR, Jacobson TA. The fats of life: the role of omega-3 fatty acids in the prevention of coronary heart disease. Arch Intern Med. 2001 Oct 8;161(18):2185–92.

Havel PJ et al. Relationship of plasma leptin to plasma insulin and adiposity in normal weight and overweight women: effects of dietary fat content and sustained weight loss. J Clin Endocrinol Metab. 1996 Dec;81(12):4406–13.

Hayashi H, Tanaka Y, Hibino H, Umeda Y, Kawamitsu H, Fujimoto H, Amakawa T. Beneficial effect of salmon roe phosphatidylcholine in chronic liver disease. Curr Med Res Opin. 1999;15(3):177–84.

Hegsted D et al. Quantitative effects of dietary fat on serum cholesterol in man. Am J Clin Nutr. 1965;17:281–295.

Hibbeln JR, Salem N Jr. Dietary polyunsaturated fatty acids and depression: when cholesterol does not satisfy. Am J Clin Nutr. 1995 Jul;62(1):1–9.

Holm T et al. Omega-3 fatty acids improve blood pressure control and preserve renal function in hypertensive heart transplant recipients. Eur Heart J. 2001 Mar;22(5):428–36.

Howard BV et al. Low-fat dietary pattern and risk of cardiovascular disease: The Women's Health Initiative Randomized Controlled Dietary Modification Trial. Journal of the American Medical Association. 2006 Feb 8;295:655–66.

Hunger JE, Applewhite TH. Reassessment of trans fatty acid availability in the U.S. Am J Clin Nutr. 1991;54:363.

Ilowite NT, Copperman N, Leicht T, Kwong T, Jacobson MS. Effects of dietary modification and fish oil supplementation on dyslipoproteinemia in pediatric systemic lupus erythematosus. J Rheumatol. 1995 Jul;22(7):1347–51.

Ioannou Y, Isenberg DA. Current concepts for the management of systemic lupus erythematosus in adults: a therapeutic challenge. Postgrad Med J. 2002 Oct;78(924):599–606.

Jain S, Gaiha M, Bhattacharjee J, Anuradha S. Effects of low-dose omega-3 fatty acid substitution in type-2 diabetes mellitus with special reference to oxidative stress—a prospective preliminary study. J Assoc Physicians India. 2002 Aug;50:1028–33.

Jenkins AB et al. Carbohydrate intake and short-term regulation of leptin in humans. Diabetologia. 1997 Mar;40(3):348–51.

Keys A et al. Serum cholesterol response to changes in the diet. Metab. 1965;14: 776–87.

Kidd PM. Attention deficit/hyperactivity disorder (ADHD) in children: rationale for its integrative management. Altern Med Rev. 2000 Oct;5(5):402–28. Review.

Knopp RH et al. One-year effects of increasingly fat-restricted, carbohydrate-enriched diets on lipoprotein levels in free-living subjects. Proc Soc Exp Biol Med. 2000 Dec;225(3):191–9.

Kobayashi N et al. Effect of altering dietary omega-6/omega-3 fatty acid ratios on prostate cancer membrane composition, cyclooxygenase-2, and prostaglandin E2. Clin Cancer Res. 2006 Aug 1;12(15):4662–70.

Kremer JM. n-3 fatty acid supplements in rheumatoid arthritis. Am J Clin Nutr. 2000 Jan;71(1 Suppl):349S-51S.

Kris-Etherton PM. Polyunsaturated fatty acids in the food chain in the United States. Am J Clin Nutr. 2000 Jan;71(1 Suppl):179S–88. Review.

Kris-Etherton P et al. Effects of dietary stearic acid on plasma lipids and thrombosis. Nutr Today. 1993;28(3):30–38.

Lean ME et al. Weight loss with high and low carbohydrate 1200 kcal diets in free living women. Eur J Clin Nutr. 1997 Apr;51(4):243–8.

Maes M, Christophe A, Bosmans E, Lin A, Neels H. In humans, serum polyunsaturated fatty acid levels predict the response of proinflammatory cytokines to psychologic stress. Biol Psychiatry. 2000 May 15;47(10):910–20.

Maes M, Christophe A, Delanghe J, Altamura C, Neels H, Meltzer HY. Lowered omega3 polyunsaturated fatty acids in serum phospholipids and cholesteryl esters of depressed patients. Psychiatry Res. 1999 Mar 22;85(3):275–91.

Malcolm CA, McCulloch DL, Montgomery C, Shepherd A, Weaver LT. Maternal docosahexaenoic acid supplementation during pregnancy and visual evoked potential development in term infants: a double blind, prospective, randomised trial. Arch Dis Child Fetal Neonatal Ed. 2003 Sep;88(5): F383–90.

Mars M et al. Leptin and insulin responses to a four-day energy-deficient diet in men with different weight history. Int J Obes Relat Metab Disord. 2003 May;27(5):574–81.

Matte, R. Position of the American Dietetic Association: fat replacers. J Am Diet Assoc. 1998;98:463–8.

Mayser P et al. Omega-3 fatty acid-based lipid infusion in patients with chronic plaque psoriasis: results of a double-blind, randomized, placebo-controlled, multicenter trial. J Am Acad Dermatol. 1998 Apr;38(4):539–47.

McCarger L et al. Dietary carbohydrate-to-fat ratio: influence on whole-body nitrogen retention, substrate utilization and hormone response in healthy male subjects. Am J Clin Nutr. 1988;49:1169–78.

Meksawan K et al. Effect of low and high fat diets on nutrient intakes and selected cardiovascular risk factors in sedentary men and women. J Am Coll Nutr. 2004 Apr;23(2):131–40.

Mickleborough TD, Murray RL, Ionescu AA, Lindley MR. Fish oil supplementation reduces severity of exercise-induced bronchoconstriction in elite athletes. Am J Respir Crit Care Med. 2003 Nov 15;168(10):1181–9. Epub 2003 Aug 6.

Mohan IK, Das UN. Oxidant stress, anti-oxidants and essential fatty acids in systemic lupus erythematosus. Prostaglandins Leukot Essent Fatty Acids. 1997 Mar;56(3):193–8.

Mori, TA et al. Dietary fish as a major component of a weight-loss diet: effect on serum lipids, glucose, and insulin metabolism in overweight hypertensive subjects. Am J Clin Nutr. 1999;70(5):817–25.

Mozaffarian D et al. Dietary fats, carbohydrate, and progression of coronary atherosclerosis in postmenopausal women. Am J Clin Nutr. 2004;80: 1175–84.

Nagakura T et al. Dietary supplementation with fish oil rich in omega-3 polyunsaturated fatty acids in children with bronchial asthma. Eur Respir J. 2000 Nov;16(5):861–5.

Nelson GJ, Schmidt PC, Kelley DS. Low-fat diets do not lower plasma cholesterol levels in healthy men compared to high-fat diets with similar fatty acid composition at constant caloric intake. Lipids. 1995 Nov;30(11):969–76.

Newbold, HL. Reducing the serum cholesterol level with a diet high in animal fat. South Med J. Jan;81(1):61–3, 1988.

Noakes M et al. Comparison of isocaloric very low carbohydrate/high saturated fat and high carbohydrate/low saturated fat diets on body composition and cardiovascular risk. Nutr Metab (Lond). 2006 Jan 11;3:7.

Nordoy A, Marchioli R, Arnesen H, Videbaek J. n-3 polyunsaturated fatty acids and cardiovascular diseases. Lipids. 2001;36 (Suppl):S127–9.

Passfall J et al. Different effects of eicosapentaenoic acid and olive oil on blood pressure, intracellular free platelet calcium, and plasma lipids in patients with essential hypertension. Clin Investig. 1993 Aug;71(8):628–33.

Peet M. Eicosapentaenoic acid in the treatment of schizophrenia and depression: rationale and preliminary double-blind clinical trial results. Prostaglandins Leukot Essent Fatty Acids. 2003 Dec;69(6):477–85.

Peyron-Caso E, Taverna M, Guerre-Millo M, Veronese A, Pacher N, Slama G, Rizkalla SW. Dietary (n-3) polyunsaturated fatty acids up-regulate plasma leptin in insulin-resistant rats. J Nutr. 2002 Aug;132(8):2235–40.

Popkin, B., et al. Where's the fat? Trends in US diets 1965–1996. Preventive Medicine. 2001;32(3): 245–54.

Prentice RL et al. Low-fat dietary pattern and risk of invasive breast cancer: The Women's Health Initiative Randomized Controlled Dietary Modification Trial. Journal of the American Medical Association. 2006 Feb 8;295: 629–42.

Rabinovitz S, Mostofsky DI, Yehuda S. Anticonvulsant efficiency, behavioral performance and cortisol levels: a comparison of carbamazepine (CBZ) and a fatty acid compound (SR-3). Psychoneuroendocrinology. 2004 Feb;29(2): 113–24.

Raper N et al. Nutrient content of the US food supply, 1909–1988. USDA Home Econ Res Rep. 50, 1992.

Reed MJ et al. Dietary lipids: an additional regulator of plasma levels of sex hormone binding globulin. J Clin Endocrinol Metab. 1987;64:1083–5.

Rennie KL, Hughes J, Lang R, Jebb SA. Nutritional management of rheumatoid arthritis: a review of the evidence. J Hum Nutr Diet. 2003 Apr;16(2): 97–109.

Rhodes LE et al. Effect of eicosapentaenoic acid, an omega-3 polyunsaturated fatty acid, on UVR-related cancer risk in humans. An assessment of early genotoxic markers. Carcinogenesis. 2003 May;24(5):919–25.

Rhodes LE, White SI. Dietary fish oil as a photoprotective agent in hydroa vacciniforme. Br J Dermatol. 1998 Jan;138(1):173–8.

Richardson AJ, Puri BK. The potential role of fatty acids in attention-deficit/hyperactivity disorder.Prostaglandins Leukot Essent Fatty Acids. 2000 Jul-Aug;63(1–2):79–87. Review.

Rivellese AA et al. Long term metabolic effects of two dietary methods of treating hyperlipidaemia. BMJ. 1994 Jan 22;308(6923):227–31.

Rivellese AA, Maffettone A, Iovine C, Di Marino L, Annuzzi G, Mancini M, Riccardi G. Long-term effects of fish oil on insulin resistance and plasma lipoproteins in NIDDM patients with hypertriglyceridemia. Diabetes Care. 1996 Nov;19(11):1207–13.

Romieu I, Trenga C. Diet and obstructive lung diseases. Epidemiol Rev. 2001; 23(2):268–87.

Romon M et al. Leptin response to carbohydrate or fat meal and association with subsequent satiety and energy intake. Am J Physiol. 1999 Nov;277 (5 Pt 1):E855–61.

Salmeron J, Hu FB, Manson JE, Stampfer MJ, Colditz GA, Rimm EB, Willett WC.

Sanders TA et al. Influence of n-6 versus n-3 polyunsaturated fatty acids in diets low in saturated fatty acids on plasma lipoproteins and hemostatic factors. Arterioscler Thromb Vasc Biol. 1997 Dec;17(12):3449–60.

Sargrad KR et al. Effect of high protein vs high carbohydrate intake on insulin sensitivity, body weight, hemoglobin A1c, and blood pressure in patients with type 2 diabetes mellitus. J Am Diet Assoc. 2005 Apr; 105(4):573–80.

Shahar E et al. Dietary n-3 polyunsaturated fatty acids and smoking-related chronic obstructive pulmonary disease. Atherosclerosis Risk in Communities Study Investigators. N Engl J Med. 1994 Jul 28;331(4):228–33.

Simopoulos AP. Omega-3 fatty acids in health and disease and in growth and development. Am J Clin Nutr. 1991 Sep;54(3):438–63.

Smith RD et al. Long-term monounsaturated fatty acid diets reduce platelet aggregation in healthy young subjects. Br J Nutr. 2003 Sep;90(3):597–606.

Smuts CM, Huang M, Mundy D, Plasse T, Major S, Carlson SE. A randomized trial of docosahexaenoic acid supplementation during the third trimester of pregnancy. Obstet Gynecol. 2003 Mar;101(3):469–79.

Stene LC, Joner G; Norwegian Childhood Diabetes Study Group. Use of cod liver oil during the first year of life is associated with lower risk of childhood-onset type 1 diabetes: a large, population-based, case-control study. Am J Clin Nutr. 2003 Dec;78(6):1128–34.

Su KP, Huang SY, Chiu CC, Shen WW. Omega-3 fatty acids in major depressive disorder. A preliminary double-blind, placebo-controlled trial. Eur Neuropsychopharmacol. 2003 Aug;13(4):267–71.

Su W, Jones PJ. Dietary fatty acid composition influences energy accretion in rats. J Nutr. 1993 Dec;123(12):2109–14.

Tamizi far B, Tamizi B. Treatment of chronic fatigue syndrome by dietary supplementation with omega-3 fatty acids—a good idea? Med Hypotheses. 2002 Mar;58(3):249–50.

Terry P, Lichtenstein P, Feychting M, Ahlbom A, Wolk A. Fatty fish consumption and risk of prostate cancer. Lancet. 2001 Jun 2;357(9270):1764–6.

Tidow-Kebritchi S et al. Effects of diets containing fish oil and vitamin E on rheumatoid arthritis. Nutr Rev. 2001 Oct;59(10):335–8.

Tomer A et al. Reduction of pain episodes and prothrombotic activity in sickle cell disease by dietary n-3 fatty acids. Thromb Haemost. 2001 Jun;85(6):966–74.

Troisi, R., et al. Trans-fatty acid intake in relation to serum lipid concentrations in adult men. Am J Clin Nutr. 1992;56:1019.

Uauy R, Hoffman DR, Mena P, Llanos A, Birch EE. Term infant studies of DHA and ARA supplementation on neurodevelopment: results of randomized controlled trials. J Pediatr. 2003 Oct;143(4 Suppl):S17–25.

Uauy R, Hoffman DR, Peirano P, Birch DG, Birch EE. Essential fatty acids in visual and brain development. Lipids. 2001 Sep;36(9):885–95.

Vergili-Nelsen JM. Benefits of fish oil supplementation for hemodialysis patients. J Am Diet Assoc. 2003 Sep;103(9):1174–7.

Volek JS et al. Effects of a high-fat diet on postabsorptive and postprandial testosterone responses to a fat-rich meal. Metabolism. 2001 Nov;50(11):1351–5.

Volek JS et al. Testosterone and cortisol in relationship to dietary nutrients and resistance exercise. Journal of Applied Physiology. 1997 Jan;82(1):49–54.

Wahrburg U. What are the health effects of fat? Eur J Nutr. 2004 Mar;43 (Suppl 1): I/6–11. Review.

Wang C et al. Low-fat high-fiber diet decreased serum and urine androgens in men. J Clin Endocrinol Metab. 2005 Jun;90(6):3550–9.

Wijendran V, Hayes KC. Dietary n-6 and n-3 fatty acid balance and cardiovascular health. Annu Rev Nutr. 2004;24:597–615. Review.

Williams MA, Zingheim RW, King IB, Zebelman AM. Omega-3 fatty acids in maternal erythrocytes and risk of preeclampsia. Epidemiology. 1995 May; 6(3):232–7.

Wolfe BM, Piche LA. Replacement of carbohydrate by protein in a conventional-fat diet reduces cholesterol and triglyceride concentrations in healthy normolipidemic subjects. Clin Invest Med. 1999 Aug;22(4):140–8.

Woodman RJ et al. Effects of purified eicosapentaenoic and docosahexaenoic acids on glycemic control, blood pressure, and serum lipids in type 2 diabetic patients with treated hypertension. Am J Clin Nutr. 2002 Nov;76(5): 1007–15.

Yamada T et al. Atherosclerosis and omega-3 fatty acids in the populations of a fishing village and a farming village in Japan. Atherosclerosis. 2000 Dec;153(2):469–81.

Zanarini MC, Frankenburg FR. Omega-3 fatty acid treatment of women with borderline personality disorder: a double-blind, placebo-controlled pilot study. Am J Psychiatry. 2003 Jan;160(1):167–9.

4

A Cheater's Overview

Before finding the Cheat to Lose Diet, both my wife and I had been suffering from major dietary boredom and burnout. Virtually every traditional diet we've tried called for the same day-in, day-out eating pattern—same calorie intake, same foods, same monotonous setup. Then we came across Joel's program, and wow, how refreshing! Over the last eight weeks, Carrie and I have together lost close to 30 pounds, but the best part is the variety of the Cheat to Lose Diet—we don't even feel like we're dieting. Not only that, but in addition to all the weekly diversity, we're able to frequently take a break from all dieting and eat whatever we want—without feeling guilty! This is a diet for normal people, and it has helped us to actually start enjoying eating and living healthy again.

Monty and Carrie R.

Grand Island, Nebraska

The Cheat to Lose Diet is one of the most effective diets I have ever been on. I consistently lost weight and inches week after week, leaving me down 20 inches and close to 20 pounds in only ten weeks! On other diets, I've always had uncontrollable cravings and would end up cheating. On the Cheat to Lose Diet, frequent cheating is a major reason why I've been able to achieve such great success! With the addition of more carbs every couple of days, I almost never feel hungry during the week. Furthermore, in the rare event that I do get a craving, I am able to easily resist, knowing that another Cheat Day where I'm able to eat literally anything I want is just around the corner.

Annette S.
Westminster, Colorado

The Cheat to Lose Diet helped me lose 10 pounds during the Priming Phase and 25 pounds total over ten weeks. Additionally, I have dropped roughly 6 inches from my love handles! With Cheat to Lose, you don't feel like you're dieting—you're living. It was a radical experience to see my weight go down another 2 pounds at the weigh-in following the Priming Phase's celebratory Cheat Day. At that point, I was more than convinced. Each and every week I was able to make consistent progress. My waist is now equivalent to what it was my junior year of high school. So many people have given me compliments and can't believe it when I tell them the basics of the program—cheat to lose weight, fast and easy. It really is that simple.

David W.
Plymouth, Massachusetts

I have been big pretty much all my life, cresting 200 pounds while still in high school. When I went off to college, my "freshman 15" was more like Herb's "freshman 55" due to high-calorie foods like pasta and pizza. On numerous occasions, I would try to starve off the pounds, eating nothing but salads and drinking green tea, but the weight crept back again and again. Starving myself was not the answer. I even tried South Beach and Atkins, but could never adopt them as a way of life—they just weren't realistic long-term solutions for me. Then I learned about Joel Marion's Cheat to Lose Diet; this is when things really began to change. In just under two months, I have lost just over 20 pounds (I have never previously experienced such rapid weight loss) while still eating the pasta and the pizza—only now as part of a strategic plan. I understand when and where I can enjoy these things, and because everything has a time and place on the Cheat to Lose Diet, I am confident that I'll be able to maintain this lifestyle for a long time to come.

Herb V.
Dover, Pennsylvania

With the prerequisites now behind us, it's time to get to the fun stuff—you know, the nitty-gritty of what this diet is all about. In this chapter, we're going to focus on two questions fundamental to any diet—how many meals you're supposed to eat each day, and how you know how much to eat at each meal—and give you the Cheat to Lose answer to both. I'm also going to give you a brief overview of the three phases of the diet, and then in chapter 6 we'll take a more detailed look into each phase, assuring that you have all the information needed to be successful during each (chapter 5 will be dedicated to the diet's most critical day—the Cheat Day). Let's begin with the overview.

As mentioned, the diet is made up of three phases: the Priming Phase, the Core Phase, and the Maintenance Phase—the last a lifestyle plan that allows you to keep the weight off for good. But before day 1 of the Priming Phase, we'll have our first unofficial Cheat Day. While kicking off a diet with a day of overfeeding may seem a bit strange, it is extremely important to ensure that you are starting the diet's initial phase with a hormonal environment primed for fat burning. By beginning with a Cheat Day, you make certain that leptin and other important hormones are up to speed, in order to get the most out of the initial three-week phase. So on the Saturday before you start the diet, it's your job to bump those levels up by being very liberal and enjoying anything you'd like. Pizza? Sure. Ice cream? Why not? BBQ ribs with a big side of macaroni and cheese? Be my guest. After the initial day's feast, it's time to get motivated, as week 1 of the Priming Phase takes on the form of a low-carb diet. While avoiding carbohydrates is certainly a poor choice for the long term (as discussed in chapter 3), the technique can be valuable when used for short periods of time. During the second week, we will reintroduce carbohydrates, but only those low on the glycemic index/glycemic load scales. Higher-GI/GL carbs, such as breads and pastas, are allowed during week 3, and the Priming Phase is concluded in celebratory fashion with the diet's first official Cheat Day. Below is a table outlining the three-week Priming Phase.

As you can see, there is a twenty-day period in which no cheating occurs. The purpose of this is twofold: one, to ensure that a strong red flag message is sent to the brain, and two, to resensitize

The Priming Phase

	Sunday	Monday	Tuesday	Wednesday	Thursday	Friday	Saturday
Week 1	Low carb	Low carb	Low carb	Low carb	Low carb	Low carb	Low carb
Week 2	Low GI/GL	Low GI/GL	Low GI/GL	Low GI/GL	Low GI/GL	Low GI/GL	Low GI/GL
Week 3	Higher GI/GL	Higher GI/GL	Higher GI/GL	Higher GI/GL	Higher GI/GL	Higher GI/GL	**CHEAT DAY**

leptin receptors (more on this in chapter 6)—both of which are necessary to get the most out of the weekly Cheat Days during the Core Phase. Also, with the way I've set things up, this will be a period of rapid progress, not stagnation. Expect to lose on average 7 and up to 12 or more pounds during these opening three weeks (and because plenty of carbs are included during weeks 2 and 3, this will be real fat loss, not temporary weight loss from water and glycogen); the difference will be noticeable in the way your clothes fit and in your appearance in the mirror. Lastly, rest assured that this is the longest you will ever go without indulging yourself while on the Cheat to Lose Diet.

After you complete the Priming Phase, you'll begin the Core Phase, which continues until you have reached your target weight. The length of this phase is obviously dependent on how much you'd like to lose. Each week of the Core Phase is set up as a mini Priming Phase. Sunday and Monday are low-carb days, low-GI/GL carb sources are reintroduced on Tuesday and Wednesday, and higher-GI/GL carbs such as breads, potatoes, and pastas are allowed on Thursday and Friday. Every Saturday, you will do both your body and mind a favor by eating the foods you crave with no remorse. During this phase, losses should continue steadily at a rate of up to 2 pounds and 2 inches weekly. Here is what each week of the Core Phase looks like:

The Core Phase

Sunday	Monday	Tuesday	Wednesday	Thursday	Friday	Saturday
Low carb	Low carb	Low GI/GL	Low GI/GL	Higher GI/GL	Higher GI/GL	CHEAT DAY

Understanding the Weekly Carbohydrate Progression

You may be wondering why we progress from a low-carb to a low-GI/GL and then to a higher-GI/GL diet during both the Priming and Core Phases, and if you're hypothesizing that it's leptin-related, you are correct. The Cheat Day and the weekly setup—everything about this diet—were designed with leptin and your body's natural feedback systems in mind. As mentioned in chapter 3, the low-carb diet is a far from optimal long-term approach to dieting due to chronically low insulin levels (and subsequently leptin levels), among other reasons. That said, when leptin levels are high, a low-carb approach will yield the quickest fat loss. This is why within the Cheat to Lose setup a low-carb approach is utilized immediately following a Cheat Day. After a Cheat Day, leptin levels are at their highest, so we're able to get away with limiting carb intake, as the body is still sensing that everything is "normal." Then, as levels start to drop, carbohydrates of the low-GI/GL variety are reintroduced. The additional calories and carbohydrate will help bump falling leptin levels back up to baseline, ensuring that the body is still sensing that everything is okay. After the short low-GI/GL period, the body will begin to adapt once again, and this time we use higher-GI/GL carbohydrates to send an even stronger signal to the brain. Higher-GI/GL carbs induce a greater insulin response, and as previously mentioned, insulin has strong ties with leptin. By manipulating carb intake in this manner (in addition to the Cheat Day), we "trick" the body into thinking we're not dieting, which allows us to lose fat at an optimal rate each and every day of the diet.

Once you've reached your target weight, it's time to maintain the progress you've made. While still technically part of the diet, the Maintenance Phase isn't really a diet at all. Instead, it's a lifestyle plan with *less structure* and *more food*—while still helping you maintain your weight loss. Because you worked with your body instead of against it throughout the course of the Cheat to Lose Diet, you protected your metabolism, instead of destroying it as with other commercial diets. You won't have to live in a state of caloric restriction for the rest of your life to maintain your weight loss; you'll just need to follow a few simple guidelines—

guidelines that you've gotten so accustomed to over the course of the Core Phase that they've become a natural part of the way you live. And that's what the Maintenance Phase is all about—living and enjoying life.

So there you have it—the three phases of the diet in a nutshell. Again, we'll be outlining each phase in more detail in just a bit, so if you have questions, rest assured they will be answered shortly.

When Do I Eat?

Let's talk about the first of the two fundamental questions that I spoke of in the beginning of the chapter: how many meals should you be eating each day? As if all the dieting mistakes we've already talked about weren't enough, here we have another biggie—the idea that less is better. Recall the time you asked a coworker why she wasn't eating lunch and she replied, "I'm trying to drop a few pounds." Or how about the time you found yourself boasting to a close friend or significant other about how you made it all the way until 6 p.m. before eating something that particular day? We've all had these experiences. It's funny how we associate dietary success with eating very little, skipping meals, and depriving ourselves, when in fact such techniques have never been successful. Plenty of individuals have given that approach an honest try, and after a few weeks of less-than-mediocre results, they revert back to their old habits. If the approach worked, they would have continued with it, but no one wants to sacrifice without being rewarded eventually. Ignoring hunger and going prolonged periods of time without nourishment does nothing but kill your metabolism and hasten the delivery of that ugly red flag message to the brain. If falling leptin levels, plummeting concentrations of fat-burning hormones, and a metabolism with the speed of a tortoise are what you're after, the "skip breakfast and lunch diet" will have you well on your way to such an outcome. But if you're looking to save your precious metabolism while dieting, believe me, deprivation isn't going to be the answer.

On the Cheat to Lose Diet, you will be eating often throughout the day—every few hours or so. Breakfast, lunch, and dinner will be staples, and in addition to the standard three meals, several ample-sized snacks will be on the daily menu. I chose this frequent-feeding approach for a number of reasons. First, and most important, there is the issue of leptin and metabolism. I cannot overemphasize the point that *every* single aspect of this diet has been set up with leptin and your body's natural feedback systems in mind. Frequent feedings help to stabilize our friend leptin, and thus metabolism, by providing the body with nutrients throughout the day. If a single day of fasting is enough to cause serum leptin to hit rock bottom, you can probably guess that skipping meals and going extended periods of time without sustenance isn't exactly going to help you in your quest to shed unwanted body fat.

Also, frequent feedings allow for a better utilization-to-storage ratio of a given caloric intake. Meaning, all else being equal, if one individual consumes 2,000 calories split over two meals and another individual consumes the same 2,000 calories split over five meals, the former would store most of those calories, while the majority of calories ingested by the latter would be more readily used for energy. The reason is there is an upper limit on the number of calories the body can utilize during the average digestion period. The first person is consuming 1,000 calories per sitting, much more than the body is able to utilize at one time, so many of those calories are stored. This doesn't seem like such a big deal, as you might figure the stored calories would just be released and used as energy at some point during the day anyway, but unfortunately the body will be reluctant to "give up" these calories, as leptin levels aren't optimized as a result of the infrequent feedings. So, as you can see, larger, sporadic meals really are a double whammy when it comes to effective weight loss.

Before moving on to the next point, I want to briefly touch on another way frequent feedings help to increase energy expenditure, and that is through something known as the thermic effect of feeding, or TEF. TEF is just a fancy name for the amount of energy burned during the digestion process. With frequent feedings, your body's digestive engine is fired up numerous times each day, and that constant stimulation keeps your metabolic furnace ablaze.

The second, major reason for enjoying the frequent-feeding approach is craving control. It's not likely that you'll find yourself hungry during the day, because just as your last meal or snack has worked its way through the digestive process, it's time to eat again. This makes adherence to the diet *a lot* easier. You'll also be considerably less likely to overindulge during one of your scheduled meals, as you'll never have that "Man, I'm starving!" feeling that arises when you haven't eaten all day.

Last, frequent feedings aid in the maintenance of muscle tissue while dieting, not only through the stabilization of leptin, but also by providing a steady flow of nutrients to the muscle tissue over the course of each day. When you eat only one or two meals daily, muscle tissue is "starved" for hours upon hours—certainly not the ideal situation if lean body mass preservation is the goal.

Meal Frequency: A Comparison	
Frequent Feedings	**1-2 Meals/Day**
• Preserve lean body mass	• Starves muscle tissue
• Curb hunger	• Promotes cravings
• Utilize ingested calories	• Leads to most ingested calories being stored
• Increase the thermic effect	• Discourages the burning of additional calories
• Stabilize leptin and metabolism	• Causes leptin to plummet and metabolism to crash

As a general rule, strive to eat every three hours or so. That said, it's not the end of the world if your hunger guides you to a time frame a tad longer or shorter.

How Much Can I Eat?

Now that we know how many meals and snacks you're going to consume each day, let's discuss the second question: how do you know how much to eat at each meal? Once again, the idea that less is better is not ideal. This mind-set causes many a dieter to drastically undershoot his or her calorie needs, a scenario that, as mentioned in chapter 2, results in a metabolic mess and a good amount of lean tissue loss to boot. Obviously, we want the complete opposite: optimal fat loss while maintaining as much calorie-burning, physique-defining muscle tissue as possible. The only way to obtain such an outcome is through *moderate* calorie restriction. Don't be alarmed by the term *restriction;* while you will be consuming slightly fewer calories, you won't have to sacrifice quantity be-

When to Eat

Sample Daily Timeline

7:00 a.m.	breakfast
10:00 a.m.	mid-morning snack
12:30 p.m.	lunch
3:00 p.m.	mid-afternoon snack
6:00 p.m.	dinner

cause of it. In fact, you'll likely be eating *more* than you previously were as a result of the better, healthier food choices you'll be making. For instance, your average fast-food joint can easily pack 500 calories into a relatively small burger, while a plate chock-full of colorful, flavorful foods like chicken breast, broccoli, onions, zucchini, and rice totals less, with a quantity that is much more satisfying. Quantity without the calories—that's what Sunday through Friday is all about.

Both calorie-counting and portion-control methods have been successfully used by dieters in the past to answer the "how much" question. While the former method is thought to be the gold standard due to its precision, the latter, when used correctly, can be just as effective while being a heck of a lot more practical. Precision in this instance is overrated, as some deviation in caloric intake from day to day (as is experienced with the portion-control method) is actually beneficial to "keep the body guessing," so to speak. As you are already well aware, the body is the king of adaptation, and varying caloric intake from day to day is one way to aid in the stalling of the adaptation process.

One popular approach to the portion-control method is the "plate method," an approach in which a plate of standard size (usually an 8-inch plate for men and a 6-inch one for women) is divided by imaginary lines into several sections and those sections are filled with foods from various food groups. While the method promotes a balanced approach to nutrition and does account for gender differences, it does not account for the obvious difference in size that can occur between members of the same sex. Take, for example, a 6'3" male with a large frame and another male standing 5'8" with a small frame: with the plate method, both of these individuals will consume about the same amount of calories at each sitting, and therefore each day. Needless to say, the 6'3" individual's caloric needs are much greater than those of the 5'8" individual. What ends up happening is the smallest individuals eat more than they need, the largest much less, and only a very small percentage in the middle actually consume the appropriate amount of calories. The approach is entirely too cookie-cutter to be effective.

A much better approach is to use your hand as a reference for determining portion size. People of *larger* stature eat *larger* portions due to their proportionally *larger* hand size. Similarly, *smaller*, more petite individuals consume *smaller* portions and fewer calories as a result of their hands being on the *smaller* side. This is the approach that we will be using. But first, let's understand where our portions are coming from. Within the foods we eat, there are three primary nutrients from which we obtain our daily energy—protein, carbohydrates, and fat. These are known as the macronutrients. We have discussed the latter two extensively, but the first has only been mentioned in passing up to this point. With diets centered around the limitation of fat and carbohydrates, protein tends to get lost in the background at times; however, that doesn't mean that its value is less than that of fat or carbs. Protein is our unsung hero. In fact, the macronutrient is so important, we'll be including a portion of it with every meal and snack.

Protein serves several functions within the body, the most commonly noted of which is the maintenance and repair of various bodily tissues. Many people will argue that only a small amount of dietary protein is needed to carry out the aforementioned function; however, there are other reasons beyond tissue repair and maintenance to make protein a staple macronutrient in any dietary regime. First, protein has the greatest thermic effect of feeding. If you recall, TEF is the amount of energy required to digest the food we eat; therefore, a protein-rich diet will actually allow you to burn more calories *through eating*. And if that's not a

Protein—Dangerous?

Over the course of the last few years, you've probably read a newspaper or magazine article or tuned in to a television special report claiming that high-protein diets are "hard on the kidneys" or contribute to osteoporosis. Being that I'm advocating a fair amount of protein with this diet, it's probably best that I take a few minutes to clear up some of the misinformation regarding protein intake and health.

One of the supposed dangers associated with high protein intake is renal (kidney) dysfunction; however, there has not been one study using healthy individuals as subjects that shows this to be the case. In fact, the argument is based on research conducted on subjects who already had some sort of renal disorder. If high protein intake really caused renal failure, there would be a nationwide epidemic among athletes, bodybuilders, and high-protein dieters; instead, it's unheard of.

Another is the idea that high protein intake leaches calcium from bones and contributes to osteoporosis. When analyzed, the amount of calcium excreted is so incredibly small that a single glass of milk per week could replace the amount several times over. Considering that milk, cottage cheese, and other dairy products are generally staples in any high-protein diet, this is really an overblown issue.

A third argument against protein-rich diets is that they put individuals at greater risk to develop kidney stones. Again, there are no studies to prove that high protein intake causes kidney stone formation, and once again, this *may* be an issue only if you previously had a kidney stone in that it *may* put you at greater risk for recurrence. You see the word *may* there several times, as this would be the case only if the previous stone was of the uric acid variety—which accounts for only 20 percent of all stones. Having said that, unless you have a family history or some sort of preexisting medical condition that makes you susceptible to uric acid stone formation, this too is a nonissue.

All in all, the idea that a diet rich in protein is dangerous for normal, healthy people is one that has been extremely exaggerated. Don't believe everything you read or hear!

good enough reason (although I can't imagine it not being), protein ingestion stimulates the secretion of the hormone glucagon, a hormone with antagonistic properties to those of insulin. In other words, glucagon helps to minimize insulin's negative effects on fat storage. Additionally, glucagon also inhibits the activity of several other enzymes playing a role in fat storage. Simply put, a diet rich in protein leads to less fat storage and greater fat loss.

Now, let's get back to appropriate portion sizes for both protein and carbohydrates. This is the rule: a portion of protein on the Cheat to Lose Diet should be equal in size and thickness to the palm of your hand. This could be a chicken breast or a turkey breast; a steak, a hamburger, or some other form of beef; various finfish or shellfish; a pork or lamb chop; a venison steak; fresh ham; or even something as simple as eggs or cottage cheese. We'll measure carbs a little differently, this time equating a portion of carbohydrate to the size of your clenched fist. This could be a bowl of oatmeal or oat bran; a side of lentils or other beans; a couple of new potatoes; a single sweet potato or yam; carrots, corn, pasta, or rice; an apple, an orange, a peach, or a pear; kiwi, diced melon, grapes, strawberries, or mixed berries; a slice or two of whole-grain bread; a whole-wheat tortilla; or again, something as simple as light yogurt or no-sugar-added applesauce.

What about green vegetables? Yes, green veggies do contain carbs, but these vegetables are 90 percent fiber and you'd have to eat a truckload of them to total a significant amount of calories. Not only that, but they have the highest concentration of vitamins, minerals, and phytochemicals of any food out there. We aren't going to put a limit on green veggies such as lettuce, green beans, broccoli, asparagus, and spinach; freely add them to any meal or use them along with a big glass of water to curb late-night or between-meal cravings. Additionally, a comprehensive list of "free" vegetables that may be consumed at any time in unlimited amounts is given in chapter 6.

Last is fat, which doesn't require that same portion measurement, the reason being that if your protein choice already contains a good amount of fat, there is no need to add additional fat to the meal. Having said that, there are many different cuts of red meat with varying fat content, so which do you choose? Honestly, there is no reason to be extremely cautious when picking out a steak or a roast; just choose something that looks decently lean and trim any visible fat before cooking. If you're going with ground beef, however, I'd recommend 95 percent lean, as it will yield just the right amount of fat per portion. But what if your protein source is very lean, such as chicken breast or certain types of fish or shell-fish? This is where the art of adding fat comes in. Fat can be easily added to a meal in any number of ways; here are just a few.

- Add olives, olive oil, ground flaxseed, and/or nuts to salads.
- Add butter or olive oil to greens and other veggies.
- Enjoy a side of avocado or guacamole.
- Enjoy a modest handful of nuts as an appetizer, a side, or part of a snack.
- Spread almond or other nut butter on celery as an appetizer, a side, or part of a snack.
- Consume a tablespoon or two of almond or other nut butter for dessert.
- Add flavor to veggies, poultry, and other foods with reduced-fat shredded cheese.
- Supplement your meal with fish oil.

Obviously, you'd add fat through only one of these tactics in a single meal. You wouldn't dress your salad with olive oil, enjoy a side of avocado with your protein source, *and* finish the meal off with a handful of nuts; you'd do one of the three. If adding butter or olive oil to greens, please note: the greens are free, the butter or olive oil is not. Along the same lines, anytime you add fat to a meal or snack, remember that you're substituting for the amount of fat in the average portion of red meat or other fat-containing protein source (9 to 11 grams for small individuals, 12 to 14 grams for those with a medium build, and 15 to 17 grams for people of larger stature), so don't go bonkers with the oil, butter, cheese, or nuts. Once you become accustomed to the amount of fat in a particular source, it's okay to eyeball amounts used, but initially, it is recommended that you take a few seconds to look at the label and use the above gram recommendations.

We will be consuming a portion of protein with every meal, but things are not so uniform for the other two macronutrients. Some meals will include one portion of carbs, some two, and some none depending on the day. Likewise, in some meals we will include fat, and in others we will steer away from its use. You will learn about this shortly, as the exact setup for low-carb days, low-GI/GL days, and higher-GI/GL days will be thoroughly outlined in chapter 6. Additionally, plenty of sample menus and recipes suitable for each day are provided in Parts II and III to make things even easier. But before we do that I'm going to address the most important day of the diet—the Cheat Day.

References

Belko AZ et al. Effect of energy and protein intake and exercise intensity on the thermic effect of food. Am J Clin Nutr. 1986 Jun;43(6):863–9.

Cho S et al. The effect of breakfast type on total daily energy intake and body mass index: results from the Third National Health and Nutrition Examination Survey (NHANES III). J Am Coll Nutr. 2003 Aug;22(4):296–302.

Farshchi HR et al. Beneficial metabolic effects of regular meal frequency on dietary thermogenesis, insulin sensitivity, and fasting lipid profiles in healthy obese women. Am J Clin Nutr. 2005 Jan;81(1):16–24.

Farshchi HR et al. Decreased thermic effect of food after an irregular compared with a regular meal pattern in healthy lean women. Int J Obes Relat Metab Disord. 2004 May;28(5):653–60.

Farshchi HR et al. Deleterious effects of omitting breakfast on insulin sensitivity and fasting lipid profiles in healthy lean women. Am J Clin Nutr. 2005 Feb;81(2):388–96.

Karst H et al. Diet-induced thermogenesis in man: thermic effects of single proteins, carbohydrates and fats depending on their energy amount. Ann Nutr Metab. 1984;28(4):245–52.

Kinabo JL, Durnin JV. Thermic effect of food in man: effect of meal composition, and energy content. Br J Nutr. 1990 Jul;64(1):37–44.

Kirt TR. Role of dietary carbohydrate and frequent eating in body-weight control. Proc Nutr Soc. 2000 Aug;59(3):349–58. Review.

Louis-Sylvestre J et al. Highlighting the positive impact of increasing feeding frequency on metabolism and weight management. Forum Nutr. 2003;56: 126–8. Review.

Nair KS et al. Thermic response to isoenergetic protein, carbohydrate or fat meals in lean and obese subjects. Clin Sci (Lond). 1983 Sep;65(3):307–12.

Schutz Y et al. Postprandial thermogenesis at rest and during exercise in elderly men ingesting two levels of protein. J Am Coll Nutr. 1987 Dec;6(6): 497–506.

U.S. National Library of Medicine and National Institutes of Health. Protein in diet. Medline Plus Medical Encyclopedia. 2003.

Westerterp-Plantenga MS. High protein intake sustains weight maintenance after body weight loss in humans. Int J Obes Relat Metab Disord. 2004 Jan;28(1):57–64.

After dropping 12 pounds during the Priming Phase, I was a little apprehensive about implementing an eat-whatever-I-want Cheat Day each week during the Core Phase. Six weeks later, down a total of 13½ inches (4 on my waist!) and just over 20 pounds, I think it's safe to say I no longer have those concerns. The Cheat to Lose Diet is an amazing tool—a fun, easy way to lose weight. Coming into the diet, I didn't really know what to expect, but after seeing results like these, I'll never attempt to lose weight another way.

Chris M.

Toronto, Ontario, Canada

The Cheat to Lose Diet is the only truly livable diet that I've come across. At fifty-three, I've been on my fair share of diets, and never before have I been able to lose weight so quickly and easily, let alone while cheating on my diet so frequently! In only eight weeks' time, I was able to exceed my goals by dropping 27 pounds and four pants sizes. I feel better, look better, and have more energy than I've had in years. Thank you!

Jeff G.
Cupertino,
California

I had never been on a diet before, but after having my son I knew I needed to do something to lose my postpregnancy weight. Fortunately, I came across Cheat to Lose. In just ten weeks I was able to lose all of the weight I'd gained and then some; I'm actually now fitting into jeans that I haven't been able to wear for the last three years! And just as Joel prescribed, every week I cheated big, enjoying anything I felt like eating—and each week, the scale read less and less. With the Cheat to Lose Diet, both the Cheat Day and week-to-week results kept me motivated. I'm enjoying being healthier while still being able to eat foods I'd never be able to eat on other diets on a weekly basis.

Young-ha K.
Daejoen, South Korea

5

The Cheat Day

Dieting in general has always been intimidating to me. While I have tried many, including the Zone and various low-carb approaches, all the rules and regulations were always too cumbersome, difficult, and time-consuming. Then I read about Cheat to Lose, and for once a dieting approach actually looked fun! Throughout the course of the diet, I put the Cheat Day to the test with everything from pizza to lasagna to McDonald's, but each and every week, the scale reflected less and less—it was hard to believe! Over the course of eight weeks, I was able to effortlessly lose 18 pounds. The Cheat to Lose Diet has opened my eyes to the simplicity of becoming and remaining healthy. This is something I will continue for the rest of my life.

Scotty B.

Ottawa, Ontario, Canada

Although diet books don't typically have climaxes, the excitement surrounding the Cheat Day is sure to make this chapter atypical in that regard. Although I could more or less sum up the chapter with one word, *eat*, there are a few rules I'd like to go over to ensure that you obtain the most benefit from your daylong dietary feast.

Rule Number 1: Eat the Foods You Crave Without Feeling Guilty

This is the numero uno rule of the Cheat Day. I trust that after reading chapter 2, you understand how putting this rule into action will in no way hinder fat loss, but instead will accelerate it. Even after being armed with this scientific knowledge, you may have some reservations about being completely free to eat whatever you want. After all, the idea that a day of dietary cheating can actually hasten progress is, at least at this time, a radical concept. When you come upon your first official Cheat Day, having made substantial progress during the Priming Phase, you may be tempted to play it safe and be conservative with the foods and amounts you consume. *Don't*. While it's natural to think that by doing so you'll be preserving your recent fat loss, in actuality you're only hindering your long-term progress.

A classic example of this can be found in what happened to a woman I worked with who came to me about six months after her first child was born. She was having difficulty losing the weight she had put on during pregnancy and was still roughly 25 pounds heavier than before. She had tried several dietary tactics to rid herself of the unwanted body fat, but nothing seemed to work. After our initial consultation, I had her start the Priming Phase. At its end she was down a very noticeable 9 pounds. At that point, she continued with the Core Phase for the next several weeks; however, her progress was far from optimal. I asked how closely she was adhering to the strict portion of the diet, and she said she hadn't deviated at all from the foods I recommended. I was perplexed as to what the problem might be, and after manipulating several other variables to no avail I finally thought to ask her to outline what a typical Cheat Day looked like for her. What I got in response showed that she was cheating herself out of her Cheat Day! I asked her why she was being so conservative, and she replied that she was so pleased with the 9-pound drop during the Priming Phase that she didn't want to "mess it up." Like many others, after experiencing the rapid progress of the Priming Phase, she thought an all-out Cheat Day would put her back at square one. It's no wonder her progress was less than optimal. Despite religiously adhering to the strict portion of the diet, she failed to properly carry out the diet's most vital day—the Cheat Day. Needless to say, I informed her that her recent lack of progress was likely a result of her *lack of cheating*. Still a bit nervous about gaining back lost weight, she put her trust in me and began eating more liberally on her Cheat Day. Immediately her weekly progress doubled, and before long she found herself back within a few pounds of her prepregnancy weight, both feeling and looking great.

To have success on this diet, you really have to throw out everything you've been told previously and take a leap of faith. If you do, you will be extremely pleased with the results. However, if you hold on to the doctrine of the past, you're going to end up shortchanging yourself, plain and simple.

The Cheat Day is not just a day or a meal randomly thrown into the diet to make the diet more appealing; it's not something that is simply "allowed," nor is it an "extra" of some sort. It is a critical aspect of the diet and is absolutely vital to your success. You *must* cheat, and do so liberally, to achieve optimal fat loss. If you wake up with blueberry pancakes on your mind, by all means fire up the griddle. Top them with butter, maple syrup, whipped cream, more blueberries—whatever you want; nothing is off-limits. If later in the day you get an urge for pizza, pay a visit or make a call to your favorite pizzeria. Enjoy. That's what the Cheat Day is all about.

Rule Number 2: Start Your Cheat Day When You Normally Wake Up on Saturday

This is another important guideline, and it's one that 90 percent of people will break unless expressly told otherwise. After all, it's human nature to push the envelope and see what we can get away with, especially when it's not specifically stated in the rules. Take it from someone who's been there. That's right, within the aforementioned 90 percent was an individual whom you've all grown very familiar with by now—yours truly. Since I was the initial tester of virtually all my theories, you have the luxury of learning from all my past mistakes, and Cheat Day was certainly no exception. During my preliminary runs, I would get a little overanxious when it came to the much-anticipated Cheat Day. Come 12 a.m., I'd begin. After a few hours of indulgence, I'd allow myself several hours of sleep and then get up to continue with my day of dietary defiance. As one could probably guess, my literal interpretation of the term *day* in this instance didn't exactly result in the fat loss I was looking to achieve. Sure, I made progress, but it wasn't *optimal* progress. And the thing was, I *knew* I was limiting my fat loss by starting the cheat session prematurely each week, but at the same time I would justify doing so because, well, starting the night before at the peak of my nocturnal cravings was a heck of a lot easier than resisting those cravings and waiting until morning! Bottom line, anytime you feel as though you're trying to get away with something on the Cheat Day, you're probably pushing your limits a tad too much. While you are encouraged to cheat on this diet, trying to cheat the cheating system itself is not recommended!

Along those same lines, don't set the alarm for an abnormally early time in an attempt to tack on a few additional hours to your weekly cheat. Doing so will only be to your detriment, and for a number of reasons. First, let's consider the effect of this type of behavior on sleep and your hormones. Setting the alarm for a very early hour both causes you to wake up abruptly and limits the amount of quality sleep you're getting on what is probably the most critical night of each week. Waking up sleep-deprived causes a number of negative things to occur inside of you hormonally; to make a long story short, it basically throws everything out of whack. On the morning of the Cheat Day, an optimal hormonal start is one in which hormones are relatively stable and normalized—clearly not the scenario present when you wake up at an unusually early hour. I once had a college-age client whose class schedule was set up so that on most days he could sleep in until 10 a.m. or later. However, on Cheat Days, he'd set the alarm for 6 a.m. in anticipation of consuming all the food he'd been craving over the last few days. Needless to say, the hormonal situation created by doing this each Cheat Day was far from ideal, as the time he was awakening on Saturday differed so much from what his body was used to throughout the rest of the week. A word to the wise: if you're used to getting up well into the morning hours, there's no need to rise with the sun on your Cheat Day. Similarly, if you typically sleep in on the weekends to recuperate from a taxing workweek, by all means, sleep in on your Cheat Day as well. The whole point of the Cheat Day is to let things happen naturally. A natural awakening ensures that hormones and hormonal patterns will be more or less normalized, stable, and relatively uninterrupted—the optimal setup for the Cheat Day.

A second reason waking up extremely early on your Cheat Day is a poor choice is that it makes the day as a whole less enjoyable. Yes, you may get a few extra hours to chow down, but the overall quality of the day will be sacrificed. This also ties in with the hormonal issues mentioned above. When you wake up naturally, appetite-stimulating hormones are heightened, and breakfast, especially a cheater's breakfast, will be welcomed by the body, both physically and mentally. Conversely, if you wake up sleep-deprived, with its associated hormonal environment, your appetite isn't all that stimulated. This leaves the start of your Cheat Day, and subsequently the rest of that day, less appealing and enjoyable. I don't know about you, but when my Cheat Day rolls around, I want to make sure I enjoy it. Quality over quantity. And believe me, you'll have plenty of time to eat everything you want by simply waking up naturally anyway.

Rule Number 3: Don't Stuff Yourself

Here is one rule that many a dieter will fall victim to. Simply because you're encouraged to consume foods on your Cheat Day that are typically off-limits during the week doesn't mean you *have* to eat every last thing available to you. If you're dining out and become full, wrap the rest up and finish it later. If you're not hungry, don't force yourself to eat because you feel this is your only shot for another week and you have to make it count. Enjoy the day; it's your day. Eat to the point of satisfaction, not discomfort. Once satisfied, wait until you are at least semi-hungry again and then plot your next meal. Being stuffed and extremely uncomfortable all day long is anything but enjoyable and desirable—certainly not the intended purpose of the Cheat Day.

Rule Number 4: Don't Skip Meals Because You're Holding Out for a Single Feast

This is a critical mistake, unfortunately made all too often. What happens is this: you get invited to a party, plan a big family dinner, or have some sort of social outing to attend on your Cheat Day, and in anticipation of the big event you hold out or save your appetite for later in the day. Don't do this. Studies have shown that prolonged periods of overfeeding are needed to boost leptin levels back to baseline and to restore that fat-burning hormonal milieu we talked about so extensively in chapter 2. A *day* of cheating is necessary; a couple of hours or a single meal just isn't long or intense enough to clear the red flag message being sent to the brain all week. To obtain optimal results, you need to eat throughout the day. Sure, it's okay to give yourself a cushion of a couple of hours before attending a party or sitting down to dinner, but as the inverse to Cheat Day Rule Number 3, there should never be a time during which you are hungry yet not eating. Do not, I repeat, *do not* actively deny your body what it is asking for. If you're not hungry, wait until you are, but if you *are* hungry, *don't* wait.

Rule Number 5: Don't Plan

You may have noticed many of the rules mentioned in this chapter contradict those you'll be asked to follow throughout the week; here's another one. While it will be strongly recommended that you plan meals ahead of time for regular days, the Cheat Day is a day in which it is preferred that you simply go with the flow. Many times, especially for a first Cheat Day, dieters will meticulously plan each and every food they intend to consume. Oftentimes, however, upon awakening they discover the foods they had originally planned to eat aren't foods they're craving. Problem is, the fridge and cupboard are already stocked. Which brings me to my next point: don't go shopping during the week for foods to consume on your Cheat Day. Why? For one thing, as just mentioned, you don't really know what you're going to crave most until you wake up the morning of your Cheat Day and let the day play out. Second, we've all heard the recommendation to avoid visits to the grocery store while hungry, as you're much more likely to buy items you don't really need or for that matter even want. When you're hungry, especially when dieting, everything looks appetizing. Before you know it, you're zipping to the checkout counter with an entire cart of goodies, most of which you'll never even tap into come Saturday. Additionally, you just subconsciously made the next several days leading up to your Cheat Day harder because you now have massive amounts of off-limits foods right at your fingertips to tempt you. It's a heck of a lot easier to overcome a craving when what you're craving is not readily accessible. Also, consider the aftermath: because you went shopping for your Cheat Day midweek, not only did you spend too much money and unnecessarily torture yourself with seemingly overwhelming temptation for several days, but now you're dealing with the fact that you've overstocked and didn't even touch half of what you bought. Once again, you have highly tempting food items lying around the house—but now while you're trying to stay on the low-carb portion of the diet week.

Trying to plan out your Cheat Day ahead of time will likely just cause a myriad of problems to arise. So simply wake up and go with the flow; you'll enjoy the day more this way and at the same time save yourself needless headaches.

Rule Number 6: Avoid Excessive Alcohol Consumption

Enjoying a cold beer or a glass of wine is perfectly fine on your Cheat Day; what you need to be careful of, however, is *excessive* alcohol consumption. While one or two drinks won't appreciably affect progress, excessive alcohol intake certainly will. Studies have shown that alcohol consumption acutely decreases blood levels of leptin, which is exactly the opposite of what we're trying to accomplish by overfeeding on the Cheat Day. So if you're drinking to the point of intoxication, know you've considerably surpassed the acceptable amount. In all honesty, I'd prefer that alcohol be completely avoided if possible, as it's an area where many push the envelope, but I'd be lying if I said that beer or wine with a meal every so often on your day off would cause you ill effects. Just be sure to limit yourself to one or two drinks max for the day.

Some Closing Words

The Cheat Day should be an all-around enjoyable day. At times, and understandably so, all of us can get a little too anxious or excited and unknowingly get in our own way. This chapter outlines rules to prevent that from happening and to ensure two things: that you're obtaining the greatest physiological benefit from your Cheat Day and that you're enjoying your day as much as you should be. With that in mind, let's begin to take a deeper look at the three phases of the diet in our next chapter.

References

Calissendorff J et al. Is decreased leptin secretion after alcohol ingestion catecholamine-mediated? Alcohol & Alcoholism. 2004 Jul-Aug;39(4):281–6.

Dammann G et al. No significant effect of acute moderate alcohol intake on leptin levels in healthy male volunteers. Addict Biol. 2005 Dec;10(4):357–64.

Rojdmark S et al. Alcohol ingestion decreases both diurnal and nocturnal secretion of leptin in healthy individuals. Clin Endocrinol (Oxf). 2001 Nov;55(5): 639–47.

6

The Cheat to Lose Diet

I absolutely love this diet! With the help of Cheat to Lose, I've dropped 34 pounds and 6 inches on my waist in just eight weeks! As someone who is very into sports and resistance training, I had always steered away from dieting for fear of losing strength and performance due to a lack of carbs and calories. But because this diet allowed for plenty of both, I decided to give it a shot. In the end, I'm healthier and more agile, and amazingly, my strength hasn't decreased at all; in fact, it's gone up! The only thing I've lost is my gut and a bunch of unwanted body fat.

Jack B.

Hollywood, Florida

I started the Cheat to Lose Diet about one year after my second child was born. Unlike after my first child, I was having a hard time losing the weight I had put on during pregnancy. Despite keeping to a very strict diet, I hadn't made much progress in literally months, so I decided to give something different a try. That something different was Joel's Cheat to Lose Diet. During the three-week Priming Phase alone I was able to drop 3 inches from my waist and just about another 3 from my hips! Wow! That was more progress in three weeks than I had experienced during the previous three months. Before long, I was fitting back into my old clothes again and am currently feeling the best I've felt in years!

Lisa U.
Tarknok, Hungary

The Cheat to Lose Diet is one of the coolest things I've ever had the opportunity to do. To be honest, it's fantastic. I'm a fitness model who needs to stay in top condition year-round, and the Cheat to Lose Diet has proved to be the easiest, most effective, most realistic means for me to do so. The most exciting part is I get to revisit my childhood days of putting away mounds—scratch that—boxes of glorious cereal on a weekly basis, all while maintaining 4 percent body fat and getting more work now than ever before. For me, the Cheat to Lose Diet has become a way of life—a diet that I can live with.

John R.
Long Island, New York

I have been considered overweight my whole life. At twenty-four, I knew I didn't want to be "the fat girl" for the rest of my life, and I knew I needed to make a change. So I tried dieting. I tried Weight Watchers and South Beach, and while they worked for a short while, I was not able to stick with them for any length of time—they just weren't realistic for me for the long term. With Cheat to Lose, however, not only was I able to stick with the diet, but over the course of ten weeks, I lost 12 percent body fat and 17 inches and even managed to gain several pounds of calorie-burning muscle and a lot of confidence. All of my clothes are baggy now and I'm actually excited about going clothes shopping! I'm finally out of plus-size clothing. Cheat to Lose is the easiest diet I've ever been on and the only one I've been able to follow through on. Knowing I'll be able to have my favorite chocolate frosted Pop-Tarts come Saturday makes sticking to the diet throughout the week an easy task.

Michelle G.
Ronan, Montana

The Priming Phase

s mentioned previously, the Priming Phase is three weeks in duration and follows this week-to-week structure:

	Sunday	Monday	Tuesday	Wednesday	Thursday	Friday	Saturday
Week 1	Low carb	Low carb	Low carb	Low carb	Low carb	Low carb	Low carb
Week 2	Low GI/GL	Low GI/GL	Low GI/GL	Low GI/GL	Low GI/GL	Low GI/GL	Low GI/GL
Week 3	Higher GI/GL	Higher GI/GL	Higher GI/GL	Higher GI/GL	Higher GI/GL	Higher GI/GL	**CHEAT DAY**

As stated, there is a twenty-day period in which no cheating occurs. While a challenge, this three-week Priming Phase is absolutely critical to the success you experience during the Core Phase for a number of reasons, which we're about to explore.

Type II Obesity?

When leptin was first discovered by scientists in the mid-1990s, it was originally thought that the primary cause of modern-day obesity had been uncovered. Similar to type I diabetes, where individuals are born incapable of producing adequate amounts of insulin, obesity was hypothesized to be the result of an inability to produce enough leptin. After all, a genetic disorder in which very little or no leptin is being produced would cause the body to think it is literally always in a state of starvation, resulting in permanently slowed metabolism and increased fat storage (pretty much the ideal recipe for obesity). Medical professionals and pharmaceutical companies alike were excited at the potential development of a "leptin replacement therapy" system and a new medicinal means to control the seemingly out-of-control obesity epidemic. Unfortunately, further research showed scientists' initial hypothesis to be slightly misdirected. When analyzing blood samples of obese subjects, instead of the theorized shortage of leptin, they found an *abundance* of the hormone. In essence, what happens with leptin in obese subjects is actually very similar to what happens with insulin in type II diabetics (not type I). With a type II diabetic, there is more than enough insulin being produced, but the problem rests in the fact that the hormone is not functioning properly. This phenomenon is known as insulin resistance and occurs when insulin is no longer effectively communicating with its associated receptors. Insulin resistance is the result of years of poor nutritional habits and chronically high levels of insulin caused by consumption of insulin-spiking carbohydrates day after day. Essentially, over time, receptors build up a resistance to the hormone, rendering even the highest blood levels useless. Long-term poor dietary habits can cause a degree of "leptin resistance" to develop in overweight individuals. While there may be an abundance of leptin present (as observed when analyzing blood samples of the obese subjects mentioned above), the hormone is unable to optimally communicate with its associated receptors and therefore such high levels aren't worth a whole lot.

So what was the point of my telling you that? Well, just as insulin resistance can be reversed through dietary means, so can leptin resistance, and enhancing leptin receptor sensitivity is a major function of the Priming Phase. The diet's initial cheat-free weeks serve to jump-start leptin sensitivity to ensure that come week 4 you'll be well on your way to getting the most out of each Cheat Day and the general leptin-boosting setup of the Core Phase.

And More

A second function of the Priming Phase is to make certain that a strong red flag message is sent to the brain prior to commencing the weekly cheats of the Core Phase. When is a slice of pizza or a carton of hot french fries most satisfying? When you're already full? Of course not. These things are most gratifying when it's been hours since you've eaten and you're extremely hungry. Similarly, a surplus of calories will have the greatest physiological effect after several weeks of lower-calorie dieting, when the body is "hungry" for a metabolic boost.

A third and potentially overlooked function of the Priming Phase is to acclimate you to the three different types of days of the Cheat to Lose Diet. As mentioned previously, some days of the diet will be low-carb in nature, some low-GI/GL, and others higher-GI/GL. During the Priming Phase, an entire week is dedicated to each type of day in order to give you plenty of time to familiarize yourself with the ins and outs of each. By the time the Core Phase rolls around and the types of days shift more rapidly, the kinds of foods and meals you'll be consuming on each will have become more or less second nature.

A final function/benefit of the Priming Phase is to establish in your daily life new, healthier eating habits. It is said that it takes twenty-one days to form a new habit, and not so coincidentally that is the exact length of the Priming Phase. When twenty-one days have passed, you'll find that new habits have begun to take root. Additionally, you will be experiencing a unique sense of accomplishment, and rightfully so—you just made it through the most difficult part of the diet and can now sit back and relax knowing that it only gets easier from here.

The Day Before

So it's the day before the official start of the Priming Phase, and here's what I need you to do: eat, relax, and enjoy. This unofficial Cheat Day serves to get all those last-minute cravings out of your system before commencing the more rigid three-week Priming Phase. If there's a particular food you are going to miss dearly over the next twenty-one days, be sure to include it on today's menu. Physiologically, it is important that we start the diet with the brain sensing everything as normal, as we want to make as much progress as possible over the next three weeks. While one of the main functions of the Priming Phase is to ensure that the red flag message is sent to the brain, we still want this phase to be a period of rapid progress (which it will be), and that will happen optimally only if leptin and various other hormones are floating around at baseline levels or higher on day 1.

Ideally, this should be a memorable day in which you eat liberally and treat yourself to the foods you love most (as should every Cheat Day). Take some time to pay a visit to your favorite restaurant and order that entrée that makes your taste buds tingle. Stop off for ice cream on the way home. Have Grandma bake you her famous apple pie. Eat whatever you like and as much of it as you like (while following those same basic Cheat Day rules outlined in chapter 5). The point is to enjoy the day while setting yourself up for success over the course of the next three weeks.

Revisiting the Meal Schedule

Every day (with the exception of the Cheat Day), regardless of the phase or type of day, will follow the same basic meal schedule. As mentioned in chapter 4, you will eat often throughout the day to preserve calorie-burning muscle mass, curb hunger, and most important, stabilize leptin and metabolism. So you will be eating five times daily (three main meals and two snacks), as outlined below.

The size and composition of these five meals will differ depending on the day, so let's take a look at each type of day.

The Three Types of Days

Low-Carb Day Basics
- One portion of protein per meal/snack
- One serving of fat per meal/snack (if the protein source already contains substantial fat, it is not necessary to add additional fat)
- Zero servings of carbs per meal/snack
- "Free" veggies as desired

When to Eat	
Sample Daily Timeline	
7:00 a.m.	breakfast
10:00 a.m.	mid-morning snack
12:30 p.m.	lunch
3:00 p.m.	mid-afternoon snack
6:00 p.m.	dinner

Free Veggies

Asparagus
Broccoli
Brussels sprouts
Cabbage
Cauliflower
Celery
Collard greens
Cucumber
Eggplant
Fennel
Green onions
Leeks
Lettuce, any type
Mushrooms
Okra
Onions
Peppers
Radishes
Snow peas
Spinach
Tomatoes
Zucchini

Low-GI/GL Day Basics

- One portion of protein per meal/snack
- One serving of fat per meal/snack (if the protein source already contains substantial fat, it is not necessary to add additional fat)
- Two portions of low-GI/GL carbs with main meals (one must be fruit); one portion with snacks
- "Free" veggies as desired

Acceptable Carbohydrates on Low-GI/GL Days

- Legumes: kidney beans, black beans, black-eyed peas, lima beans, red beans, marrowfat peas, chickpeas, pinto beans, butter beans, navy beans, lentils
- Fruit: apples, oranges, apricots, peaches, pears, grapes, kiwis, mangoes, watermelon, honeydew, cantaloupe, rhubarb, plums, pineapple, papaya, grapefruit, grapes, blueberries, strawberries, blackberries, raspberries, cranberries, cherries
- No-sugar-added applesauce
- Light yogurt
- Other vegetables: artichokes, beets, pumpkin, rutabaga, squash
- Whole-grain breads: 100 percent whole wheat, pumpernickel, rye, oat bran, buckwheat, barley kernel (limit to one slice per day on low-GI/GL days)
- Other grain products: barley, brown rice, basmati, quinoa, oatmeal, oat bran, 100 percent whole-wheat tortillas (limit to one serving per day on low-GI/GL days)
- Sweet potatoes, yams (limit to one serving per day on low-GI/GL days)

Ideally, the bulk of carbs on these days should come from legumes and fruits. Additionally, there is no limit to the amount of "free" veggies you can consume. As you will see in the sample menus, however, other carbs mentioned above (oatmeal, whole-grain breads/tortillas, sweet potatoes, yams, etc.) have been included so that you never feel deprived. If you need more help, the menus given in Part II of the book will give you an even clearer picture of what a low-GI/GL day should look like.

Higher-GI/GL Day Basics

- One portion of protein per meal/snack
- One portion of higher-GI/GL carbs per meal/snack
- Minimal fat per meal/snack (be sure to choose lean protein sources)
- "Free" veggies as desired

Acceptable Carbohydrates on Higher-GI/GL Days

- Any carb source from the low-GI/GL list (limit legumes and fruit)
- Wild rice, brown rice, basmati
- Couscous
- Cornmeal
- Cereals: All-Bran, Special K, Cheerios, Fiber One, Bran Chex, bran flakes
- Pasta
- New potatoes
- Carrots, corn, peas, parsnips
- Bananas

The majority of carbs on these days should come from various grains, breads, potatoes, and pastas (again, fruit and legumes are okay, but limit their use on these days in favor of the "starchier" carbs/grains listed above). Also, given that we are limiting fat intake with each meal/snack on higher-GI/GL days, you'll want to

Acceptable Fat Choices

Dairy
- Butter
- Cheese
- Cottage cheese
- Cream

Fat-Containing Meats
- Beef
- Chicken (dark meat)
- Duck
- Lamb
- Pork

Fish
- Anchovies
- Bluefish
- Herring
- Salmon
- Mackerel
- Sardines
- Tuna

Oils
- Canola oil
- Extra-virgin olive oil
- Fish oil
- Flaxseed oil

Raw Nuts
- Almonds
- Brazil nuts
- Hazelnuts
- Peanuts (in moderation)
- Pecans
- Walnuts

Other
- All-natural peanut butter (in moderation)
- Almond butter
- Avocado/guacamole
- Eggs
- Flaxseeds (ground)

Acceptable Protein Choices

- Beef (steak, ground beef, etc.)
- Cottage cheese
- Venison
- Eggs (whole or whites)
- Finfish (salmon, haddock, mackerel, tuna, bluefish, herring, etc.)
- Fresh ham
- Lamb
- Milk protein blend (whey and casein)
- Pork (tenderloin, chop, etc.)
- Shellfish (scallops, shrimp, clams, oysters, crab, lobster, etc.)
- Skinless chicken (breast, thigh, wing, etc.)
- Turkey breast

choose lean protein sources such as chicken breast or turkey breast and avoid dark-meat chicken and anything but extremely lean cuts of red meat.

Some protein sources are also ample sources of fat and as such are included in both lists. As mentioned earlier, if your protein source already contains substantial fat, it is not necessary to add additional fat to that meal/snack. Again, always choose lean protein sources on higher-GI/GL days.

Also, you will see that peanuts and all-natural peanut butter are listed as "in moderation." This is because peanuts are a very common food allergen and chronic consumption can provoke the development of a minor food allergy and have a substantial impact on fat loss. Additionally, they are more carb-heavy than other nuts, so be conscious of your intake, especially on low-carb days.

Soy Protein: Healthful?

After looking over the list of acceptable proteins, you may have noticed that soy protein is not listed. This is not a mistake, nor is it an oversight; soy protein has been purposely left out, and I'd like to explain why. There is quite a bit of research supporting the notion that soy may not be the super health food it's sometimes made out to be. Numerous studies have linked the consumption of soy protein to decreased male hormone (i.e., testosterone) levels, sperm count, sperm production, and fertility. Studies have also shown soy to decrease thyroid output as well as HDL cholesterol (the "good" cholesterol), and it may even increase the likelihood of birth defects and below-average birth weights in newborns. On a similar note, infants fed soy-based formulas may suffer from future impaired sexual and reproductive development. These are issues that no one takes lightly; unfortunately, most people are unaware of their existence.

The problems that arise from regular soy ingestion are mostly a result of the phytoestrogens (plant estrogens, also known as isoflavones) found in soy, specifically the isoflavones genistein and daidzein. These isoflavones possess estrogenlike properties and when ingested act like estrogen in the body; while a little soy isn't anything to be concerned about, considerable soy intake on a daily basis may be. And while there are authorities on both sides of the fence (as there always are), even the American Heart Association confirms that neither the safety nor efficacy of soy isoflavone supplements has been proven. The AHA has also recently reversed its position regarding the health benefits of soy, now stating that the food has little effect on cholesterol and is unlikely to prevent heart disease. Because of the controversy surrounding soy, my personal stance and recommendation for Cheat to Lose dieters is that soy protein intake be minimized in favor of more desirable milk protein supplements (whey and casein). That said, there's no reason to become soy-phobic either; a few grams here and there or the rare consumption of a soy product is more than okay.

Don't Panic

During week 1 you will likely lose significant scale weight, while weight loss during weeks 2 and 3 will be considerably less dramatic. Because of the reintroduction of carbohydrates during week 2, it is likely that scale weight will begin to travel back up from your week 1 end. *Do not panic or get discouraged.* As mentioned in chapter 3, anytime carbohydrate intake is heavily restricted, you will initially lose substantial glycogen (stored carbohydrate in muscle tissue) and water weight. Because of the lack of carbohydrate being ingested on a daily basis, the body first turns to your muscle carbohydrate reserve for its energy needs. This results in somewhat dramatic initial weight loss, as several pounds of water will likely be lost along with at least a pound of glycogen. Then, when carbohydrates are reintroduced, the previously lost glycogen and water are restored, causing scale weight to travel back up. You are not gaining back lost fat, so do not worry. *I repeat, this does not mean you are losing progress, as you are not gaining back body fat at all.* In effect, while scale weight at the end of weeks 1 and 2 may be the same, you will have indeed lost fat during week 2. For example, you may lose 2 pounds of fat during week 2 while gaining back 2 pounds of water and glycogen; in the end, scale weight remains unchanged but measurements are down and you're looking and feeling better—and that's what's really important.

As dieters, we have become highly dependent on the scale as a measure of progress. Unfortunately, especially when carbohydrate intake is frequently changing, the number on the scale is a poor indicator. To most effectively and accurately track progress over the course of the Priming Phase, use your beginning and ending scale weight, while relying on tape measurements as your primary assessment tool throughout. At most, step on the scale once weekly at week's end. Doing so more frequently will accomplish nothing more than breaking your focus and causing unnecessary stress and worry—don't do it.

Because you are starting and ending the Priming Phase with full glycogen stores, you can rest assured that the pounds you shed by the end of the first three weeks are actually fat and not water or glycogen.

The Celebratory Cheat Day

You did it. You made it through the Priming Phase. You fought; you conquered; you prevailed. You're leaner and healthier; you feel better, look better, and have shown you've got what it takes to follow through on what you've set out to achieve. In my opinion, that calls for a celebration, and a celebration is exactly what we're going to have. Let today, the mark of a true accomplishment, be one of your most memorable on the Cheat to Lose Diet. May it be a day full of good food and good company. Have fun, stick to the very loose Cheat Day guidelines, and enjoy. You certainly deserve it.

The Core Phase

The Core Phase is the diet's main phase and begins immediately after the completion of the three-week Priming Phase. Essentially, as stated previously, each week of the Core Phase is set up as a mini Priming Phase, with the beginning of the week being low-carb in nature, midweek taking on the low-GI/GL structure, and then the latter part of the week calling for higher-GI/GL carbs. Day 7 of each and every week is a Cheat Day. Once again, here's what it looks like:

Sunday	Monday	Tuesday	Wednesday	Thursday	Friday	Saturday
Low carb	Low carb	Low GI/GL	Low GI/GL	Higher GI/GL	Higher GI/GL	**CHEAT DAY**

The only real differences between the Core Phase and the Priming Phase are that the types of days now shift more rapidly (every two days, instead of weekly) and more frequent cheating is implemented. Everything else stays the same.

During each week of the Core Phase, we combat falling leptin levels through the addition of more carbohydrate and calories every couple of days and then conclude each week with a big leptin-boosting Cheat Day. Again, it all makes perfect physiological and psychological sense. By periodically cheating on your diet, you circumvent the negative physiological side effects of calorie restriction. Each week you start fresh with baseline levels of leptin and a hormonal environment primed for burning fat, not muscle. The metabolic crash that occurs with prolonged dieting is no longer an issue, so keeping lost weight lost as you enter the Maintenance Phase of the diet won't be a problem.

I truly believe you're going to have a blast achieving awesome week-to-week progress during this phase. In fact, the general consensus has been that people don't even feel like they're dieting, and because you're not depriving yourself, I'm confident you'll agree. This is the way weight loss was meant to be achieved. Once again, you'll continue with the Core Phase until you've lost all the fat you desire to and then you'll maintain your new body with the help of the diet's final phase (which could also be called the Cheat to Lose lifestyle)—the Maintenance Phase.

The Maintenance Phase

At this point, you have reached your goal weight and it's time to maintain the wonderful progress you've made. You're going to do just that with the help of the diet's third phase.

Tracking Progress

In order to most accurately track progress, you will be taking both weekly girth measurements and scale weight readings. The locations for the various girth measurements are as follows:

Bust/chest
Waist (around the navel)
Hips
Right arm
Right thigh
Right calf

Men have the option of simply monitoring their waist measurement from week to week, as males tend to store most of their fat around the midsection (and this is where the majority of fat will be lost from). In women, however, fat loss is typically more spread out, and in order to obtain the most accurate picture of what is happening, the full array of measurements across the body needs to be taken.

For arm, thigh, and calf measurements, simply double each to account for the other limb when calculating total inches lost. For example, if your right thigh measurement has gone down one inch, it is safe to assume that your left thigh measurement has also decreased by one inch, for a total of two inches lost from both thighs.

Below are sample measurements for a female who used the Cheat to Lose Diet for six weeks:

	Starting	Week 6	Difference
Bust	38"	35"	-3"
Waist	36"	33"	-3"
Hips	38"	36"	-2"
Right arm	12"	11.5"	-.5" x 2 = -1"
Right thigh	24"	22.5"	-1.5" x 2 = -3"
Right calf	12"	11.5"	-.5" x 2 = -1"
		Total	-13"

Starting measurements will be taken the Sunday you begin the Priming Phase and then weekly measurements will be taken every Saturday thereafter first thing upon arising and before eating anything. It is of utmost importance that you measure in the same exact place, the same exact way, and at the prescribed time to ensure week-to-week accuracy. Consistency in measuring is a must; otherwise it's useless.

Also, as touched on in the "Don't Panic" section of this chapter, stay off the scale and leave the measuring tape in the drawer during the week. Expect fluctuations in water weight in response to carbohydrate manipulation and Cheat Days (and daily fluctuations in general); daily measurements mean nothing. Week-to-week measurements taken at the same time each week are all that matter; measuring the difference in these readings is the only way to ensure absolute accuracy when evaluating progress. If you choose to ignore my recommendation here, you will only end up causing yourself unnecessary stress and worry (which in turn will slow progress).

The Cheat to Lose Metabolism-Saving Effect

All throughout your time on the Cheat to Lose Diet, you did something extremely important—you protected your metabolism. This is the major downfall of most other commercial diets and dieting techniques. Regardless of the diet, all share the same problem: they call for dieters to remain in the same calorie-restricted state day after day and week after week—and no matter how you slice it, continual calorie restriction is going to adversely affect metabolism over the long term. So unless you plan on eating the same amount of food or less for the rest of your life (which is no way to live), get ready to watch the results of your sacrifice on these diets begin to slip away the minute you attempt to resume some sort of normal eating plan. Sound familiar? For many, I'm sure it does. We've circumvented this by constantly manipulating carbohydrate and calorie intake and, more important, by cheating on your diet on a weekly basis. These aspects of CTL prevented your body from catching on to the fact that you were dieting; antistarvation mechanisms never fully engaged and metabolism was safeguarded. Because of this, there are no special precautions that need be taken to prevent weight gain after coming off the Core Phase; instead, you're able to jump right into the higher-carb and -calorie nature of the Maintenance Phase without having to worry about lost fat piling back on. If you're someone who has had difficulty keeping lost weight off in the past, you now know that it's not you, and you are not doomed to be overweight for the rest of your life. Instead, because of CTL's metabolism-saving effects, you should find maintaining the progress you've made a much easier task than it has been previously.

The Cheat to Lose Lifestyle

While still technically part of the Cheat to Lose Diet, the Maintenance Phase is more a loose set of guidelines to live by than a diet per se. It is a phase of less structure, more food, and more flexibility when compared to the previous two phases, and rightly so. In essence, it is a lifestyle—a continuation of all the things you've grown accustomed to thus far, but in an even more livable format.

During this third and final phase, the basics of the Cheat to Lose Diet stay the same—frequent feedings, balanced meal composition, choosing healthy carbs and fats—while a few changes have been made to allow for more flexibility and long-term practicality. One change is that low-carb days are now a thing of the past (the only exception being the Sunday and Monday following the Core Phase's final Cheat Day—the first two days of the Maintenance Phase). This means more calories and carbs each week. Another difference is that there are no specific days set aside to implement the low-GI/GL and higher-GI/GL days. Simply because Monday is a low-GI/GL day one week does not mean that the following Monday will also be low-GI/GL. The only general guideline with respect to types of days is that you should have at least three low-GI/GL days per week. That said, how you choose to employ this guideline is completely up to you and may change week to week. This also gives you day-to-day flexibility in that if you had originally planned for a low-GI/GL day but for whatever reason decide after waking up that you'd like to enjoy some higher-GI/GL carbs, you can make the switch right then and there. Nothing is written in stone.

But what about Cheat Days? Instead of full-blown Cheat Days, we are going to use Cheat Meals while employing something known as the 90 Percent Rule. By omitting low-carb days and increasing carb-containing days, you will no longer be in a calorie-restricted state throughout the week. This means that there is no red flag message being sent to the brain, so the need for an all-out Cheat Day to combat this is no longer necessary. But there is still the occasional psychological need to indulge in "unapproved" foods (if for no other reason than these foods are part of living and enjoying life), and that's where the 90 Percent Rule comes in. The 90 Percent Rule is something that I've borrowed from my colleagues Joy Bauer and John Berardi (John is also responsible for the fantastic recipes included in the sample menus and recipe section of this book), and it works tremendously well for those looking to eat healthy while still living a normal life. In a nutshell, the rule states that 90 percent of the time you should stick to healthy food choices (Cheat to Lose–approved foods that have now more or less become part of your daily eating life), while the other 10 percent of the time you may choose other, nonapproved "cheat" foods. The rationale is that if you're making healthy food choices 90 percent of the time, what you do during the other 10 percent

Meal Replacements

Times and situations will inevitably arise in which a highly convenient, quick, and easy snack or meal is in order. During these times, the availability of a healthy meal replacement bar or shake can often be the deciding factor in whether you end up consuming the scheduled nutritious meal or instead fall victim to a lack of planning and end up making a poor food choice or skipping a meal entirely (neither of which is a good solution).

Unfortunately, the idea of a healthy meal replacement has become somewhat of an oxymoron. The protein bars and powders of old were most akin to bland shoe leather and flavored chalk, respectively, and so the public cried out for a decent-tasting, edible meal replacement. Manufacturers responded—by dumping loads of sugar and less-than-desirable fats into their product formulations. In the end, two types of manufacturers emerged: Manufacturer A, most concerned with delivering products with appealing taste, compromising on the ingredients, and Manufacturer B, most concerned with delivering quality ingredients, compromising on the taste. In time, the Manufacturer B type more or less died out, leaving nothing more than mildly protein-fortified milk-shake mixes and candy bars currently stocking nutritional supplement and grocery store shelves. While decent-tasting, these are a far cry from nutritious or healthy.

That said, there are a few lines of meal replacement products currently available that contain both the taste and the quality ingredients to allow me to comfortably recommend their use in conjunction with the Cheat to Lose Diet. One in particular is Metabolic Drive (MD) bars and shakes. MD products are in a class of their own in that their manufacturer, Biotest Laboratories, has managed to develop some of the best-tasting meal replacement products without compromising one iota on their nutritious nature. Metabolic Drive offers three different products, each of which can be implemented conveniently and effectively within the setup of the Cheat to Lose Diet: MD Complete, a complete meal replacement containing high-quality proteins, slowly digested carbohydrates, fiber, and essential fatty acids; MD Low-Carb, a low-carb, low-fat quality milk protein blend; and MD Protein-Energy Bars. MD Complete and MD Protein-Energy Bars are good as a snack or meal replacement on low- or higher-GI/GL days. MD Low-Carb can be used as the protein portion of any meal or snack on any day.

Other acceptable low-carb milk protein blends include Ultra Peptide by Xtreme Formulations and Myolean Evolution by Myogenix. Myoplex and Myoplex Lite nutrition shakes by EAS are also acceptable options; however, it is recommended that regular consumption of any soy-containing product be avoided.

While the use of any meal replacement product is not mandatory or necessary to experience success with the Cheat to Lose Diet, the addition of these products will add a degree of ease and convenience to your daily meal planning and the overall implementation of the Cheat to Lose Diet.

Here are some situations in which it's best to implement meal replacement products:

- As a midmorning or midafternoon snack
- As a quick breakfast on rushed mornings
- When working (at home or on the job)
- When available food options are limited
- Anytime when a quick and easy meal is necessary due to time constraints

---

METABOLIC DRIVE PORTION EQUATER

Metabolic Drive Complete (1 snack/meal)

Small: 2 scoops (approx. 20 grams protein, 10 grams carbs)

Medium: 3 scoops (approx. 30 grams protein, 15 grams carbs)

Tall: 4 scoops (approx. 40 grams protein, 20 grams carbs)

Note: Recommendations are based on mixing with skim milk.

Metabolic Drive Low-Carb (1 protein portion)

Small: 1 scoop (20 grams protein)

Medium: 1½ scoops (30 grams protein)

Tall: 2 scoops (40 grams protein)

Note: Recommendations are based on mixing with water.

Metabolic Drive Protein-Energy Bars (1 snack/meal)

Small: 1 bar

Medium: 1 bar

Tall: 1½ bars

For your convenience and enjoyment, Metabolic Drive smoothie recipes for all three types of days are included in the recipe section. Each delicious smoothie recipe serves as a complete meal replacement.

isn't going to significantly add to or take away from your efforts—and that's essentially true. Because Cheat to Lose calls for thirty-five meals/snacks weekly, the 90 Percent Rule gives you the flexibility of consuming three Cheat Meals each week in which otherwise "unapproved" foods may be eaten. The same don't-stuff-yourself rule from Cheat Days applies to Cheat Meals as well—enjoy, but don't abuse.

Still, though, you will inevitably have days that are close to a full-blown Cheat Day, and that's more than fine. Again, the Maintenance Phase is a long-term, realistic solution to maintaining the healthy, fit body you've achieved, and it's designed with the realization that life is full of birthdays, holidays, and other special occasions in which food is central. If you ever find you've indulged a bit too much (and if you don't at some point, you're not living properly), the resolution is simple: just revert to the Priming Phase and complete weeks 1 and 2 (the low-carb and low-GI/GL weeks). At that point, if you still want to lose a bit more fat, jump into the Core Phase for a few weeks until you're where you want to be. Once you get there, it's back to the Maintenance Phase. The dynamic nature of the diet's three phases is such that remaining fit and healthy for the rest of your life couldn't be easier.

The simple guidelines presented in this chapter have been designed with flexibility, practicality, and livability in mind. That's what the Cheat to Lose Maintenance Phase is all about—living and enjoying a healthy life.

Maintenance Cheat Sheet

- Utilize only low-GI/GL and higher-GI/GL days—no low-carb days, except for the first two days of the Maintenance Phase.

- Be sure to include at least three low-GI/GL days weekly.
- Employ the 90 Percent Rule by having three Cheat Meals weekly. Again, this does not mean a large pizza followed by a pint of ice cream—these are moderate-sized meals composed of typically off-limits foods.
- Revert to the Priming and/or Core Phases to shed holiday or vacation pounds.

References

Anderson et al. Effect of various genotoxins and reproductive toxins in human lymphocytes and sperm in Comet assay. Teratog Carcinog Mutagen. 1997;17(1);29–43.

Ashton E, Ball M. Effects of soy as tofu vs meat on lipoprotein concentrations. Eur J Clin Nutr. 2000 Jan;54(1):14–9

Atanassova N et al. Comparative effects of neonatal exposure of male rats to potent and weak (environmental) estrogens on spermatogenesis at puberty and the relationship to adult testis size and fertility: evidence for stimulatory effects of low estrogen levels. Endocrinology. 2000 Oct;141(10): 3898–907.

Barinaga M. "Obese" protein slims mice. Science. 1995 Jul 28;269(5223):475–6.

Carlsson B et al. Obese (ob) gene defects are rare in human obesity. Obes Res. 1997 Jan;5(1):30–5.

Casanova M et al. Developmental effects of dietary phytoestrogens in Sprague-Dawley rats and interactions of genistein and diadzein with rat estrogen receptors alpha and beta in vitro. Toxicol Sci. 1999 Oct;51(2):236–44

Chorazy PA et al. Persistent hypothyroidism in an infant receiving a soy formula: case report and review of the literature. Pediatrics. 1995 Jul;96(1 Pt 1): 148–50.

Chu NF et al. Dietary and lifestyle factors in relation to plasma leptin concentrations among normal weight and overweight men. Int J Obes Relat Metab Disord. 2001 Jan;25(1):106–14.

Cline JM. Effects of dietary isoflavone aglycones on the reproductive tract of male and female mice. Toxicol Pathol. 2004 Jan-Feb;32(1):91–9.

Considine RV, Caro JF. Leptin: genes, concepts and clinical perspective. Horm Res. 1996;46(6):249–56. Review.

Diamond FB Jr et al. Demonstration of a leptin binding factor in human serum. Biochem Biophys Res Commun. 1997 Apr 28;233(3):818–22.

Dillingham BL et al. Soy protein isolates of varying isoflavone content exert minor effects on serum reproductive hormones in healthy young men. J Nutr. 2005 Mar;135(3):584–91.

Dirlewanger M et al. Effects of short-term carbohydrate or fat overfeeding on energy expenditure and plasma leptin concentrations in healthy female subjects. Int J Obes Relat Metab Disord. 2000 Nov;24(11):1413–8.

Echwald SM et al. Identification of two novel missense mutations in the human OB gene. Int J Obes Relat Metab Disord. 1997 Apr;21(4):321–6.

Fine JB, Fine RM. Leptin levels in obesity. Int J Dermatol. 1997 Oct;36(10):727–8.

Flynn KM et al. Effects of genistein exposure on sexually dimorphic behaviors in rats. Toxicol Sci. 2000 Jun;55(2):311–9.

Habito RC et al. Effects of replacing meat with soyabean in the diet on sex hormone concentrations in healthy adult males. Br J Nutr. 2000 Oct;84(4): 557–63.

Haffner SM et al. Leptin concentrations and insulin sensitivity in normoglycemic men. Int J Obes Relat Metab Disord. 1997 May;21(5):393–9.

Haffner SM et al. Leptin concentrations, sex hormones, and cortisol in nondiabetic men. J Clin Endocrinol Metab. 1997 Jun;82(6):1807–9.

Halaas JL et al. Physiological response to long-term peripheral and central leptin infusion in lean and obese mice. Proc Natl Acad Sci USA. 1997 Aug 5;94(16):8878–83.

Halaas JL et al. Weight-reducing effects of the plasma protein encoded by the obese gene. Science. 1995 Jul 28;269(5223):543–6.

Hamann A, Matthaei S. Regulation of energy balance by leptin. Exp Clin Endocrinol Diabetes. 1996;104(4):293–300. Review.

Havel PJ et al. Relationship of plasma leptin to plasma insulin and adiposity in normal weight and overweight women: effects of dietary fat content and sustained weight loss. J Clin Endocrinol Metab. 1996 Dec;81(12):4406–13.

Hernandez Morin N, Perlemuter L. Leptin: a genetic solution to obesity? Presse Med. 1997 May 17;26(16):770–3.

Increased obese mRNA expression in omental fat cells from massively obese humans. Nat Med. 1995 Sep;1(9):953–6.

Irvine CHG et al. Phytoestrogens in soy-based infant foods: concentrations, daily intake, and possible biological effects. Proc Soc Exp Biol Med. 1998 Mar; 217(3): 247–53.

Jenkins AB et al. Carbohydrate intake and short-term regulation of leptin in humans. Diabetologia. 1997 Mar;40(3):348–51.

Klein M et al. Energy metabolism and thyroid hormone levels of growing rats in response to different dietary proteins—soy or casein. Arch Tierernahr. 2000;53(2):99–125.

Koutsari C et al. Plasma leptin is influenced by diet composition and exercise. Int J Obes Relat Metab Disord. 2003 Aug;27(8):901–6.

Kumi-Diaka J et al. Cytotoxic potential of the phytochemical genistein isoflavone (4',5',7–trihydroxyisoflavone) and certain environmental chemical compounds on testicular cells. Biol Cell. 1999 Sep;91(7):515–23.

Lohrke B et al. Activation of skeletal muscle protein breakdown following consumption of soybean protein in pigs. Br J Nutr. 2001 Apr;85(4):447–57.

Lonnqvist F et al. Overexpression of the obese (ob) gene in adipose tissue of human obese subjects. Nat Med. 1995 Sep;1(9):950–3.

Madani S et al. Dietary protein level and origin (casein and highly purified soybean protein) affect hepatic storage, plasma lipid transport, and antioxidative defense status in the rat. Nutrition. 2000 May;16(5):368–75.

Maffei M, Halaas J et al. Leptin levels in human and rodent: measurement of plasma leptin and ob RNA in obese and weight-reduced subjects. Nat Med. 1995 Nov;1(11):1155–61.

Nagata C et al. Inverse association of soy product intake with serum androgen and estrogen concentrations in Japanese men. Nutr Cancer. 2000;36(1):14–8.

Newbold RR et al. Uterine adenocarcinoma in mice treated neonatally with genistein. Cancer Research. 2001;61:4325–8.

Pollard M et al. Prevention of spontaneous prostate-related cancer in Lobund-Wistar rats by soy protein isolate/isoflavone diet. Prostate. 2000 Oct 1;45 (2):101–5.

Prolo P, Wong ML, Licinio J. Leptin. Int J Biochem Cell Biol. 1998 Dec;30(12): 1285–90. Review.

Relationship between insulin sensitivity and plasma leptin concentration in lean and obese men. Diabetes. 1996 Jul;45(7):988–91.

Reseland JE et al. Effect of long-term changes in diet and exercise on plasma leptin concentrations. Am J Clin Nutr. 2001 Feb;73(2):240–5.

Rohner-Jeanrenaud E, Jeanrenaud B. Central nervous system and body weight regulation. Ann Endocrinol (Paris). 1997;58(2):137–42. Review.

Romon M et al. Leptin response to carbohydrate or fat meal and association with subsequent satiety and energy intake. Am J Physiol. 1999 Nov;277 (5 Pt 1):E855–61.

Sacks FM et al: American Heart Association Nutrition Committee. Soy protein, isoflavones, and cardiovascular health: an American Heart Association Science Advisory for professionals from the Nutrition Committee. Circulation. 2006 Feb 21;113(7):1034–44. Epub 2006 Jan 17.

Scholz GH et al. Dissociation of serum leptin concentration and body fat content during long term dietary intervention in obese individuals. Horm Metab Res. 1996 Dec;28(12):718–23.

Sinha MK, Caro JF. Clinical aspects of leptin. Vitam Horm. 1998;54:1–30. Review.

Sirtori CR et al. Phytoestrogens: end of a tale? Ann Med. 2005;37(6):423–38. Review.

Smith SR. The endocrinology of obesity. Endocrinol Metab Clin North Am. 1996 Dec;25(4):921–42. Review.

Strauss L et al. Genistein exerts estrogen-like effects in male mouse reproductive tract. Mol Cell Endocrinol. 1998 Sep 25;144(1–2):83–93.

Ur E, Grossman A, Despres JP. Obesity results as a consequence of glucocorticoid induced leptin resistance. Horm Metab Res. 1996 Dec;28(12):744–7. Review.

Weber KS et al. Dietary soy-phytoestrogens decrease testosterone levels and prostate weight without altering LH, prostate 5alpha-reductase or testicular steroidogenic acute regulatory peptide levels in adult male Sprague-Dawley rats. J Endocrinol. 2001 Sep;170(3):591–9.

Whitten PL et al. Phytoestrogen influences on the development of behavior and gonadotropin function. Proc Soc Exp Biol Med. 1995 Jan;208(1):82–6.

Zhong et al. Effects of dietary supplement of soy protein isolate and low fat diet on prostate cancer. FASEB J. 2000;14(4):a531.11.

People tell us every day that we're looking more and more like the brothers of old—the healthy, fit Miguel and Armando. That's exciting, and we have Joel and the Cheat to Lose Diet to thank! In addition to the extreme simplicity of the diet, being able to get in such great shape with such a small amount of activity has been tremendous for both of us. No longer do we have to worry about spending hours in the gym. With the CTL Cardio Solution, we're in and out with plenty of time to dedicate to the many other demands of life. Collectively, we have lost 38 pounds and seven pants sizes, and together with our much improved cardiovascular health, we're both looking and feeling great!

Armando
and
Miguel P.
Reynosa,
Tamaulipas,
Mexico

The CTL Cardio Solution has been the ultimate exercise experience for me—and that's saying a lot coming from a national fitness competitor! Never before have I spent so little time in the gym and achieved such great results. In just eighteen minutes per session, I've been able to achieve a greater level of fitness than I ever have with sessions three times that length. In addition to the fitness component, my arms, abs, and butt are now tighter than ever before. It was initially hard to swallow the notion that a diet allowing me to eat all my favorite foods and a few eighteen-minute cardio sessions per week would allow me to achieve this type of condition, but the Cheat to Lose Diet has made a believer out of me!

Alena S.
New Plymouth, Taranaki,
New Zealand

7

Cheat Your Way Fit

After spending hours and hours in the gym getting relatively nowhere, I'm now making astounding progress with the Cheat to Lose Diet and Joel's eighteen-minute cardio sessions—I wish someone had told me about this earlier! At forty years old, I am now seeing muscle definition for the first time ever. The other day, someone even asked me if I was a fitness instructor. What a compliment! While I have always been on the petite side, I was carrying quite a bit of body fat on my small frame even at a size four. Cheat to Lose helped me drop back down to a zero, a size I hadn't worn in years—and with more muscle tone than ever before. With everything being low-carb nowadays, it was hard to believe I was allowed to eat things like pasta and rice on diet days, let alone things like cake and ice cream every Saturday! I couldn't be more pleased with my results.

Lynda C.

Ottawa, Ontario, Canada

Considering the average exercise bout only burns around 300 calories, exercise at first glance doesn't seem like it makes much difference. After all, what's 300 calories when a pound of fat is more than 3,000 calories? You might as well just eat a bit less and save yourself the trouble, right? Wrong. Once again, things go far beyond oversimplified addition and subtraction—the numbers don't come close to telling the whole story. The major benefit of exercise is not the caloric output (although that certainly helps), but rather the hormonal environment regular exercise creates within the body. In general, someone who is dieting who also exercises regularly will lose more fat and less muscle than someone who is attempting to achieve weight loss through dieting alone. Again, dieting alone will result in more muscle loss than dieting plus exercise, which couldn't be further from what we want. Muscle loss not only has a negative aesthetic effect, but more important, it results in slowed metabolism, which almost guarantees lost weight will eventually pile back on.

On the Cheat to Lose Diet, there are times when the body is extremely receptive to burning fat, like after a Cheat Day when leptin levels are high. Strategically timing exercise around these times, which we will do with the CTL Cardio Solution, will literally more than double the amount of progress you're able to make—it's that important. Even more important, regular exercise is a critical factor to improving long-term leptin sensitivity. When leptin sensitivity is increased, *everything* about Cheat to Lose works better and becomes even more effective.

Fear not—I'm not going to overwhelm you with hours of exercise each week. No, that would be contradictory to the whole premise of Cheat to Lose. With the CTL Cardio Solution, we make exercise fun and easy, and even find a way to "cheat" through the use of an advanced cardio technique that allows us to continue to burn calories at an elevated rate for hours and hours after we're done exercising. That's right—you'll be burning calories at an accelerated rate even if you're just relaxing on the couch or sitting behind a computer at work. We "cheat" our way to fitness by getting maximal results in minimal time. How's that for efficient?

Mixed-Intensity Training

The CTL Cardio Solution is meant to get you optimal results in the shortest amount of time. We do this by using a cardio method known as mixed-intensity training (MIT). MIT, unlike the monotonous, boring steady-state cardio in which exercisers work out at the same intensity for a designated period of time, is an exercise protocol in which you mix up the intensity throughout the workout by alternating periods of higher intensity with those of lower intensity. Research has shown this type of cardio workout to have many benefits over the traditional steady-state method, including:

- **More calories burned.** Although the difference between MIT and steady-state cardio with regard to calories burned during the exercise session is negligble, the total calories and fat burned as a result of MIT is substantially greater. This is due to increased excess post-exercise oxygen consumption (EPOC). In other words, the number of calories burned during the hours *after* an MIT bout is greatly increased due to a prolonged increase in oxygen consumption. This means you'll burn more calories by just sitting there after an MIT workout! With moderate-intensity, steady-state cardio, EPOC is minimal, and metabolism quickly returns to baseline following the exercise session.

- **Greater fat loss.** It makes sense that a workout that burns more calories will yield greater fat loss, but just how much greater? Well, one particular study from the journal *Metabolism* compared an MIT-type program with endurance / steady-state cardio over a fifteen-week period and found that the MIT group experienced nine times the fat loss of the steady-state group! Other studies have reported similar findings.

- **Greater fitness.** When comparing MIT to steady-state, MIT is the clear winner in improving your level of fitness and conditioning. While steady-state cardio only substantially improves your aerobic capacity (for slow-paced activities), numerous studies have shown MIT to improve both aerobic and anaerobic fitness levels (the ability to excel at both slower- and faster-paced activities). Furthermore, MIT has been shown to improve aerobic capacity even more than steady-state cardio.

By now, it should be obvious that MIT is the way to go to make the most of your time, accelerate fat loss, and quickly improve your level of fitness—which is exactly why the CTL Cardio Solution is based on MIT principles.

The CTL Cardio Solution

As mentioned, I'm not going to overwhelm you with hours of exercise each week. In fact, the CTL Cardio Solution is only eighteen minutes in duration, and you'll only perform it three or four times weekly. With this type of workout, we don't waste time—we get in, take care of business, and then enjoy the fat-loss benefits of elevated metabolism for the rest of the day, while actually accomplishing other things instead of spending hours in the gym. The workouts are short and concentrated, leaving you with a feeling of accomplishment, but they're also fresh and won't lead to burnout. At the beginning of each workout, you know that in less than twenty minutes you'll be finished, and that's a great motivator. No more hour-long cycling sessions while staring at the person on the treadmill in front of you. Instead, these sessions are lively and enjoyable. Below is an outline of the eighteen-minute workout:

Interval 1: 2 minutes light, 2 minutes hard
Interval 2: 2 minutes light, 2 minutes hard
Interval 3: 2 minutes light, 2 minutes hard
Interval 4: 2 minutes light, 2 minutes hard
Cool-down: 2 minutes very light

If you imagine a scale of 1 to 10, with 10 being maximal effort and 1 being hardly any effort, the "light" portion of the interval should be in the 3 to 4 range (what brisk walking feels like in most cases) and the hard portion of the interval should be in the 7 to 8 range (when you can't talk easily). Obviously no one is capable of doing a full-blown sprint for two minutes, but the hard portion of the interval should be very challenging and at a pace that really makes you work for those two minutes. Push yourself. Once you complete the hard and light portions of the interval, immediately begin the next interval—in other words, move the entire eighteen minutes. Also, keep in mind where you are starting. Your level of fitness may differ from someone else's, so base your pace on your own feeling of effort and exertion, and not anyone else's. Before you know it, you'll be increasing your speed and will love that you're able to do more in the same amount of time; it's a very rewarding feeling.

As far as mode of exercise is concerned, walking/running is preferred and requires no equipment if you're doing it outside, but other modes such as the treadmill, elliptical trainer, stationary cycle, stair stepper, and rower are also acceptable.

The first two days after the cheat (Sunday and Monday), leptin levels are high and the body is primed to burn fat, so you'll want to conduct a workout on each of these days. If you're feeling ambitious, you can perform two sessions on Sunday to really take advantage of this state (both morning and afternoon/evening sessions). The final session of the week should be conducted on Thursday or Friday, as leptin once again is getting a bump from the higher-GI/GL carbs. So that's one or two sessions on Sunday, one on Monday, and one on either Thursday or Friday, for three or four sessions per week. Perform these workouts in the mornings if possible to take full advantage of an entire day of heightened metabolism, but if that's not feasible, afternoon sessions will work fine.

Also, anytime you'd like to get some slower-paced, recreational activity in (perhaps taking a walk with your spouse, or participating in a sport), feel free to do so. Sunday or Monday would be a great day to plan these types of activities to take advantage of the leptin boost (really, you'll find that the fat melts right off when you stay active on these two critical days). And if you enjoy longer jogs, adding one or two per week is fine. Just be sure to get in the three or four sessions of the CTL Cardio Solution prescribed previously. Any other activity you'd like to add, by all means go right ahead. You can even add another session of the CTL Cardio Solution if you're feeling ambitious.

Get NEAT

The acronym NEAT stands for non-exercise activity thermogenesis, which is just a fancy way of saying calories burned through non-exercise-related activity. For example, we've all heard that taking the stairs is a better option than riding the elevator (even fidgeting can increase NEAT). But there are many other ways you can increase metabolism throughout the day. Form habits that promote a more physically active lifestyle. You know what they are; we all do. Just move more. Anyone can walk a little more each day, and while standing on the bus instead of sitting may seem insignificant at first, each day adds up, and before long you'll find that your goals are approaching faster and faster.

References

Bahr R et al. Effect of feeding and fasting on excess postexercise oxygen consumption. Appl Physiol. 1991 Dec;71(6):2088–93.

Bahr R et al. Effect of intensity on excess postexercise O2 consumption. Metabolism. 1991;40(8):836–41.

Bergman BC et al. Respiratory gas-exchange ratios during graded exercise in fed and fasted trained and untrained men. J Appl Physiol. 1999 Feb;86(2):479–87.

Borsheim E, Bahr R. Effect of exercise intensity, duration and mode on postexercise oxygen consumption. Sports Med. 2003;33(14):1037–60. Review.

Chu NF et al. Dietary and lifestyle factors in relation to plasma leptin concentrations among normal weight and overweight men. Int J Obes Relat Metab Disord. 2001 Jan;25(1):106–14.

Dengel DR et al. Effects of weight loss by diet alone or combined with aerobic exercise on body composition in older obese men. Metabolism. 1994 Jul;43(7):867–71.

Diboll DC et al. Cardiovascular and metabolic responses during 30 minutes of treadmill exercise shortly after consuming a small, high-carbohydrate meal. Int J Sports Med. 1999 Aug;20(6):384–9.

Dyck DJ. Leptin sensitivity in skeletal muscle is modulated by diet and exercise. Exerc Sport Sci Rev. 2005 Oct;33(4):189–94. Review.

Frank LL et al. Effects of exercise on metabolic risk variables in overweight postmenopausal women: a randomized clinical trial. Obes Res. 2005 Mar;13(3):615–25.

Gullstrand L. Physiological responses to short-duration high-intensity intermittent rowing. Can J Appl Physiol. 1996 Jun;21(3):197–208.

Gutin B et al. Effects of exercise intensity on cardiovascular fitness, total body composition, and visceral adiposity of obese adolescents. Am J Clin Nutr. 2002 May;75(5):818–26.

Haluzik M et al. Effect of aerobic training in top athletes on serum leptin: comparison with healthy non-athletes. Vnitr Lek. (Czech.) 1999 Jan;45(1):51–4.

Ishigaki T et al. Plasma leptin levels of elite endurance runners after heavy endurance training. J Physiol Anthropol Appl Human Sci. 2005 Nov;24(6): 573–8.

J Sports Med Phys Fitness. 1999 Dec;39(4):341–7.

Kondo T et al. Effect of exercise on circulating adipokine levels in obese young women. Endocr J. 2006 Apr;53(2):189–95.

Koutsari C et al. Plasma leptin is influenced by diet composition and exercise. Int J Obes Relat Metab Disord. 2003 Aug;27(8):901–6.

Kraemer RR et al. Leptin and exercise. Exp Biol Med (Maywood). 2002 Oct;227(9):701–8. Review.

Lakka TA et al. Leptin and leptin receptor gene polymorphisms and changes in glucose homeostasis in response to regular exercise in nondiabetic individuals: the HERITAGE family study. Diabetes. 2004 Jun;53(6): 1603–8.

Lee YS et al. The effects of various intensities and durations of exercise with and without glucose in milk ingestion on postexercise oxygen consumption. J Sports Med Phys Fitness. 1999 Dec;39(4):341–7.

Niklas BJ et al. Exercise blunts declines in lipolysis and fat oxidation after dietary-induced weight loss in obese older women. Am J Physiol. 1997 Jul;273 (1 Pt 1):E149–55.

Phelain JF et al. Postexercise energy expenditure and substrate oxidation in young women resulting from exercise bouts of different intensity. J Am Coll Nutr. 1997 Apr;16(2):140–6.

Reseland JE et al. Effect of long-term changes in diet and exercise on plasma leptin concentrations. Am J Clin Nutr. 2001 Feb;73(2):240–5.

Rodas G et al. A short training programme for the rapid improvement of both aerobic and anaerobic metabolism. Eur J Appl Physiol. 2000 Aug;82(5–6): 480–6.

Schabort EJ et al. The effect of a preexercise meal on time to fatigue during prolonged cycling exercise. Med Sci Sports Exerc. 1999 Mar;31(3):464–71.

Smith J et al. The effects of intensity of exercise and excess post-exercise oxygen consumption and energy expenditure in moderately trained men and women. Eur J Appl Physiol. 1993;67:420–5.

Steinberg GR et al. Endurance training partially reverses dietary-induced leptin resistance in rodent skeletal muscle. Am J Physiol Endocrinol Metab. 2004 Jan;286(1):E57–63.

Tabata I et al. Effects of moderate-intensity endurance and high-intensity intermittent training on anaerobic capacity and VO2max. Med Sci Sports Exerc. 1996 Oct;28(10):1327–30.

Tabata I et al. Metabolic profile of high intensity intermittent exercises. Med Sci Sports Exerc. 1997 Mar;29(3):390–5.

Tomlin DL, Wenger HA. The relationship between aerobic fitness and recovery from high intensity intermittent exercise. Sports Med. 2001;31(1):1–11. Review.

Tremblay A et al. Effect of intensity of physical activity on body fatness and fat distribution. Am J Clin Nutr. 1990 Feb;51(2):153–7.

Tremblay A et al. Impact on exercise intensity on body fatness and skeletal muscle metabolism. Metabolism. 1994 Jul;43(7):814–8.

Tremblay A, Doucet E. Influence of intense physical activity on energy balance and body fatness. Proc Nutr Soc. 1999 Feb;58(1):99–105. Review.

Unal M et al. Investigation of serum leptin levels and VO2max value in trained young male athletes and healthy males. Acta Physiol Hung. 2005;92(2):173–9.

Yoshioka M et al. Impact of high-intensity exercise on energy expenditure, lipid oxidation and body fatness. Int J Obes Relat Metab Disord. 2001 Mar;25(3):332–9.

8

Cheating
Q and A

The Cheat to Lose Diet is the easiest dieting approach I've ever taken on. The weekly setup and Cheat Day provide plenty of variety to satisfy every taste and avoid boredom. Furthermore, I truly believe this is a diet that literally anyone can have success with. After dropping 10 pounds during the Priming Phase, my results for the first few weeks of the Core Phase were not as good as I'd expected. I contacted Joel and he instructed me to drop the higher-GI/GL days and instead go with a three-day/three-day low-carb/low-GI/GL schedule. The next week was a great week, and that one simple switch has kept the results coming consistently, week after week. If you're not experiencing the expected results, please, give one of the tweaks mentioned in this chapter a try! Stick with it; if necessary, take a few weeks to find what works best for you—the rest of your life will thank you for it.

Deborah B.

Marion, Massachusetts

On the Cheat to Lose Diet, I lost 15 pounds during the first three weeks and over 30 pounds in ten weeks! For years, I had struggled immensely with dieting and losing weight, and had begun to lose faith in my ability to stick to any sort of dietary regimen. Then I discovered Cheat to Lose. This is the only diet I've ever been able to stick with! The weekly Cheat Days keep me on track during the week and allow me to regularly enjoy foods I'd never be able to consume on other diets. They are what make this diet possible for me. They are the reason Cheat to Lose is not simply a diet, but rather a lifestyle. This is maintainable; everything else I have tried is not. Additionally, I'm now fitting into pants and shirt sizes that I haven't worn for years, my confidence has heightened, and my energy levels have improved dramatically.

William T.
Hayward, Wisconsin

I am healthy, fit, and full of confidence. I don't feel fat. Instead I feel attractive and like the woman I know I am. Over the last twelve weeks, I have lost over 25 pounds and 30 inches. My body fat has decreased by nearly 15 percent. For the first time in a very long time, I look in the mirror and am pleased with what I see. Three months ago I was not able to make these statements. After years of trying to sort through nutritional misinformation, I met Joel and he shared with me the principles of the Cheat to Lose Diet. Suddenly, everything became clear. I feel as though I finally get it. And what's even better is I feel as though I've been equipped with all the necessary tools to keep this up for a lifetime. This diet has changed me from the outside in. It's maintainable, it's livable, and it works.

Electra S.
Mechelen,
Belgium

Without the outlet of a weekly Cheat Day, I'd never be able to stick to a diet—and to know that my Saturday feast is actually helping get the weight off makes this diet even more remarkable. In just ten weeks, I was able to reach my goal of losing 30 pounds. Without Cheat to Lose, I simply would not have been able to do it. Now, on the Maintenance Phase, I'm living and enjoying being healthier while still eating a wide variety of foods, including all my favorites. Before, sticking with a diet for more than a few days was a struggle. Now, I'm confident this is something I'll be able to continue for a lifetime.

Phillip K.
Burlington City, New Jersey

Now that we've discussed all three phases of the diet, I'd like to take some time to share with you some of the most frequently asked questions I've received from Cheat to Lose dieters along with comprehensive answers to each. Some of these questions may already have occurred to you, while others may not arise until you find yourself in a similar situation; nevertheless, the vast majority are likely to come up at some point, and this chapter will allow you to quickly and easily navigate any troubled waters.

What if cheating seems to result in a one-step-forward, one-step-backward phenomenon?

For a very select group (less than 10 percent of those who embark on the Cheat to Lose Diet), eat-whatever-you-want Cheat Days will not be the most advantageous cheating approach. If three weeks into the Core Phase you are not achieving the expected results, you may fall into this category. In this rare case, don't panic or worry. This does not mean that the diet or periodic cheating will not work for you—it will, and a simple tweak has fixed and will fix the problem nearly every time. You have three options, any of which will likely correct things and have you progressing as you should.

One option is to alter the nature of your Cheat Days from the all-out approach to one of more controlled composition. You can do this simply by limiting fat intake while concentrating on consuming mostly protein and carbohydrates—lots of high-glycemic-index/low-fat carbohydrates. So although this designates things like pizza or your typical fast-food meal as off-limits, there are plenty of other fun, satisfying options to choose from. For instance, fat-free Fig Newtons, pasta, bagels, breads, raisins, grape juice, potatoes, baked potato chips, baked tortilla chips and salsa, animal crackers, low-fat ice cream or nonfat frozen yogurt, low-fat Pop-Tarts, low-fat graham crackers, low-fat cookies, rice, and pretzels are all still fair game during your Cheat Day and with no limitation on amount. Again, the vast majority will have no problem whatsoever with regular Cheat Days and will even experience the best results with that type of approach, but for a select few the more controlled approach outlined above may be a better option.

Now, if you're someone who'd rather not give up the unrestricted nature of your Cheat Day, there are other options. One is to space your Cheat Days out a little further. So instead of two days each of low carb, low GI/GL, and higher GI/GL and cheating every seventh day, you'd go with three days apiece and cheat every tenth day. This makes things a little less uniform, as each subsequent Cheat Day would fall on a different day of the week, but it is an option that has worked quite well for some.

The final option would be to cut out the higher-GI/GL days completely and go with three low-carb days followed by three lower-GI/GL days while still cheating with the all-out approach every seventh day.

Again, the approach you choose is more a matter of personal preference than efficacy, so go with the one that makes you feel most comfortable. Whichever tweak you decide to employ, it should prove to get you right on track, experiencing the expected results.

In addition to one of the above tweaks, keep a tight rein on your portion sizes, especially carbohydrate portions. Also, it is a good idea to strive to be extra active on the first couple of days after your Cheat Day.

What if I have a social event or a dinner to attend on a day other than Saturday? Can I switch my Cheat Day?

People have lives, and that means that there will inevitably be times when moving your Cheat Day to another day is desirable. Have no worries—the Cheat to Lose Diet recognizes the need for flexibility and practicality, and with a simple adjustment or two the Cheat Day can easily be switched to a different day of the week to accommodate a special occasion. Let's say, for example, your birthday falls on a Thursday and you'd like to celebrate on that specific day. No problem—simply go with the diet as planned for the beginning portion of the week (two low-carb days followed by two low-GI/GL days) and then cheat on Thursday. On Friday, restart the cycle but add an extra low-carb day and an extra low-GI/GL day; by the following Thursday you're back on track with the prescribed higher-GI/GL days and are on schedule once again for your regular Saturday Cheat Day. It looks something like this:

Sunday	Monday	Tuesday	Wednesday	Thursday	Friday	Saturday
Low carb	Low carb	Low GI/GL	Low GI/GL	**CHEAT DAY**	Low carb	Low carb
Low carb	Low GI/GL	Low GI/GL	Low GI/GL	Higher GI/GL	Higher GI/GL	**CHEAT DAY**

If the day of the special occasion instead falls in the beginning of the week, say Sunday, adjust by adding another higher-GI/GL day before the Cheat Day, to hold you over, and then drop a higher-GI/GL day from the following week to get yourself back on schedule.

Sunday	Monday	Tuesday	Wednesday	Thursday	Friday	Saturday
Low carb	Low carb	Low GI/GL	Low GI/GL	Higher GI/GL	Higher GI/GL	Higher GI/GL
CHEAT DAY	Low carb	Low carb	Low GI/GL	Low GI/GL	Higher GI/GL	**CHEAT DAY**

I could outline specific alteration recommendations for special occasions falling on each day of the week, but I don't think that is necessary. From the previous two examples, you should have a pretty good feel for the simple changes that need to be made to make things work. And while what you come up with may differ slightly from what I would recommend, in the grand scheme of things any minor difference isn't going to matter.

Note: In these cases, take your scale weight and measurements on the morning of the Cheat Day, whatever day that may be, instead of the usual Saturday measurements.

What if I'd like my permanent Cheat Day to be Sunday instead of Saturday? I generally have family over every Sunday afternoon, and I think having my Cheat Day on this day would be best for me.

This is more than okay and a very easy switch. Have your week begin with Monday and end with Sunday and you're good to go.

Are there any long-term negative health effects that I should be concerned about with the regular indulgence of the Cheat to Lose Diet?

I can understand this concern, but let's think about this logically. You'll be eating much, much healthier six out of seven days of the week, which is going to result in improved health. Not only that, but the Cheat to Lose Diet is going to assist you in shedding pounds of unwanted fat. When you conclude the Core Phase, you're going to be carrying considerably less body fat, which will result in improved health. Additionally, the exercise component of this diet will have you improving health through markedly increased physical activity. Basically, there are far too many improvements occurring to have a single day of dietary cheating negate them. So the answer is no, I would not be concerned with any long-term negative health effects, but instead would expect to see an immense improvement in overall health as a result of your following the Cheat to Lose program.

What about diabetics or those with cardiovascular disease? Is this diet safe for them?

For anyone with the above health issues, it is best to gain control over them before beginning a program such as Cheat to Lose. Consult with your doctor to see if this diet is for you at this time and always, *always* follow his or her advice.

Pass on the Equal?

There is much controversy surrounding non-nutritive sweeteners with regard to their safety and possible adverse health effects, and specifically in relation to dieting and their possible negative effects on fat loss. That said, available research does not validate either of these concerns. In 2002, over twenty years since the food additive was approved by the FDA, a comprehensive review of all aspartame research to date concluded that aspartame is indeed safe when consumed by normal humans in acceptable amounts. How do you know what is "acceptable"? Acceptable Daily Intakes (ADIs; amount of a particular non-nutritive sweetener that a person can safely consume every day over a lifetime without risk) have been established for all approved non-nutritive sweeteners, and amounts ingested through normal dietary consumption of products containing these sweeteners do not come close to exceeding the established ADIs. Furthermore, in its 2004 position paper, the American Dietetic Association gives its stamp of approval for consumers to safely enjoy a range of non-nutritive sweeteners.

But what about the effect of these sweeteners on weight loss? Some will argue against the use of non-nutritive sweeteners, as consumption may lessen dietary adherence by causing dieters to crave other sweets. While one 2004 study gave merit to this theory, this is not supported by other research analyzing the use of aspartame as part of a weight-control program. Further, by that argument, you'd expect those taking this stance to also recommend avoiding fruits and anything else both sweet and extremely healthful—but they're not, leaving a huge inconsistency in the argument. Although sounding initially plausible, the theory simply does not pan out. In everything I have seen, the exact opposite has been true—the use of non-nutritive sweeteners *increases* dietary adherence by giving individuals a no-calorie outlet to satisfy the occasional sweet craving. Non-nutritive sweeteners provide a great alternative to sugar-laden beverages and other counterproductive sweet products and further lessen the temptation of resorting to such products to satisfy a sweet craving.

The research on aspartame and weight control, too, supports this view, including a long-term study from researchers at Harvard Medical School analyzing aspartame's impact on weight loss and long-term maintenance of lost weight. Over a nineteen-week period, study participants regularly consuming aspartame lost more weight than those abstaining from its use. Moreover, the aspartame group was able to better maintain lost weight over a two-year follow-up period when compared to the non-aspartame group. This, along with other research, supports the notion that when used in conjunction with a weight-control program, aspartame may have beneficial effects on weight loss. This is most likely a result of increased dietary adherence.

So what does this mean for you and the Cheat to Lose Diet? Unlike some others, I do not recommend the complete avoidance of non-nutritive sweeteners for either safety or weight-loss reasons, as a comprehensive look at the research supports neither. That said, if you choose to consume beverages sweetened with aspartame or other non-nutritive sweeteners, please do so in moderation as a treat and as needed. Any products containing a non-nutritive sweetener will still give rise to insulin, so do not abuse their use. If using packets, limit use to one at a time. Additionally, water, for many reasons, is still the best source of hydration and should constitute the majority of liquid you drink on a daily basis.

I'm still a little anxious about an entire day of dietary indulgence. Can't I just have a single Cheat Meal?

Not if you want to lose fat at an optimal rate and/or get any physiological benefit from your cheating. The whole purpose of the Cheat to Lose Diet's cheat sessions is to produce high levels of leptin and increased metabolic activity so that you're able to consistently lose fat week after week. A single meal will not send a strong enough signal to the brain nor boost leptin significantly; for this to happen, you need to up carbs and calories over an extended period of time. Research shows that a single day of overfeeding will accomplish this, which is why Cheat Days, not single meals, are prescribed. Trust the diet and the prescription; it takes a bit of faith at first, but your steadily decreasing waistline will thank you.

Do you recommend the use of any "damage control" supplements for the Cheat Day?

While others may recommend the use of insulin-mimicking supplements such as alpha-lipoic acid (ALA or r-ALA) for use with Cheat Meals or the like, I am of the opinion that such supplements only interfere with the natural hormonal upregulation that we are trying to produce with the Cheat Day. My recommendation: skip the supplements and let your body naturally respond to the increase in food intake.

I'm a vegetarian/vegan; can I still do this diet? What alterations do I need to make, if any?

Yes, you can absolutely still be part of the Cheat to Lose community. You'll just need to be a little more creative with your food selections to ensure you are getting enough protein. For meals in which you do not consume a portion of protein directly (because of the absence of meat), go with tofu (in moderation) and increase the legume and/or nut content of the meal, as both contain a fair amount of protein. Metabolic Drive bars and shakes may also prove to be helpful, especially Metabolic Drive Low-Carb, which can be easily subbed for the protein portion of any meal.

References

American Dietetic Association. Position of the American Dietetic Association: use of nutritive and nonnutritive sweeteners. J Am Diet Assoc. 2004 Feb;104(2):255–75.

Aspartame. Review of safety issues. Council on Scientific Affairs. JAMA. 1985 Jul 19;254(3):400–2.

Bertorelli AM, Czarnowski-Hill JV. Review of present and future use of nonnutritive sweeteners. Diabetes Educ. 1990 Sep-Oct;16(5):415–22. Review.

Blackburn GL et al. The effect of aspartame as part of a multidisciplinary weight-control program on short- and long-term control of body weight. Am J Clin Nutr. 1997 Feb;65(2):409–18.

Blackburn GL. Sweeteners and weight control. World Rev Nutr Diet. 1999; 85:77–87. Review.

Butchko HH et al. Aspartame: review of safety. Regul Toxicol Pharmacol. 2002 Apr;35(2 Pt 2):S1–93.

Kanders BS et al. An evaluation of the effect of aspartame on weight loss. Appetite. 1988;11 Suppl 1:73–84.

Rolls BJ. Effects of intense sweeteners on hunger, food intake, and body weight: a review. Am J Clin Nutr. 1991 Apr;53(4):872–8.

I'm a university student, and fitting proper nutrition into my schedule had always been a problem. With the Cheat to Lose Diet, however, I was able to eat healthy without having my diet completely consume my life. The Cheat Day also provided a nice social outlet that dieting in the past didn't offer. I could plan things for weekends very easily and without guilt. It all fit into the structure of the diet! Because of Cheat to Lose, I was able to lose just over 20 pounds of fat and almost 5 inches from my waistline, and if I can do it, anyone can.

Robert M.

Edmonton, Alberta, Canada

In twelve weeks, the Cheat to Lose Diet has helped me lose 26 pounds and 6 percent body fat (10 pounds in the Priming Phase alone). Dieting no longer feels like dieting. The variety is something I have not found with any other approach and makes this diet one I feel I can maintain for the rest of my life. This is the first time I've lasted twelve weeks at anything! The results of this experience have been so invigorating, I'm now confident I can achieve any goal I set out to accomplish—and that's exactly what I plan to do!

Corey F.

Omaha, Nebraska

9

Staying on Track

As a firefighter and a paramedic, I have a very hectic schedule—I work twenty-four-hour shifts and live three hours from my job. Still, I found it easy to plan for my eating on this diet. By implementing the planning tips Joel provided, I was able to easily consume all meals and always had the appropriate foods ready to go. Once you get the general pattern of eating down, everything else is a breeze and the diet becomes second nature. In addition to helping me lose close to 25 pounds, CTL has helped me gain confidence and the realization that I am the one in control of my weight and health. Because I am also a competitive weight lifter (with various weight classes), I sometimes had to switch to the Maintenance Phase of the diet in preparation for a meet, as I was actually losing weight too quickly on the Core Phase! But despite having to move down several weight classes, my strength has gone up and I'm competing at an even higher level. This has never been the case on any other diet I have tried!

Malinda B.

Killeen, Texas

Plan, Plan, Plan

Like with anything else, effective planning is key to your success on the Cheat to Lose Diet. Eating three meals a day plus snacks may seem a bit overwhelming at first (especially if you're only used to eating one or two), but with proper planning it becomes both extremely easy and enjoyable. Additionally, it's much more likely that you'll make a poor food choice in the absence of planning, so it's always best to cover your bases ahead of time. Should you find yourself caught up in the busyness of life, having something healthy available for your next scheduled meal won't be an issue.

To ensure success and to avoid being stuck in a position where you are forced to make a less-than-desirable meal selection, I recommend doing three things ahead of time: planning weekly menus, shopping, and cooking (in that order).

- **Plan weekly menus.** It's best to find some time on Friday or Saturday to plan the menu for the upcoming week. Be sure to take into consideration your schedule and where you will be (this is the major reason to plan—so that you're never in a position where what you need is not available). To make things easier for you, we have included many weeks of sample menu plans to assist you. You can certainly follow these plans to the letter if you wish, but they are equally useful as a starting place to develop your own meal plans.

As you plan, jot down a shopping list of items you'll need to prepare the meals of your weekly menu. Realize, too, that no plan is set in stone; you can adjust later according to your schedule and any special circumstances that may arise (including simply being in the mood for something other than what you originally planned).

- **Shop.** Once you have your meal plan for the week in place, you'll need to go shopping for any items you may not currently have in the house. Buying your groceries before the week begins will allow you to cook in advance for additional convenience.

- **Cook.** There are a few ways to cook in advance, including weekly, twice weekly, and daily. Personally, I like to go with the middle of the three options, but let's quickly review all three. With the weekly option, you'd spend a few hours on Saturday or Sunday doing all the major cooking for the week. You'd then store the food in the fridge to be quickly and easily reheated at the designated mealtime within your plan. The twice-weekly option is very similar, with the exception that you'll cook two times each week (once at the beginning of the week and then again midweek). I like this option best because it's still highly convenient but doesn't have you eating week-old food on Thursday and Friday. Yet another option is to prepare all meals for the day in the morning, but this may not be realistic for those getting the kids to school and then rushing off to a busy day at work. If you are someone who is generally home throughout the day, however, this is a great approach. You also may want to prep all daytime meals beforehand and cook dinner fresh most evenings; it's really up to you so long as the approach you choose doesn't leave you unprepared.

Conquer with Convenience

The more convenient things are for you, the easier the implementation of the Cheat to Lose Diet will be. The use of Metabolic Drive bars and shakes, the ease of reheating a precooked meal, the inclusion of quick and easy snacks (protein cookies, protein pudding, parfaits)—all these things are built into the diet's recommendations to make things easier for you.

Additionally, when cooking in advance, you can make things even more convenient for yourself by storing your prepared cuisine in single-meal containers. This way, the only thing you need to do to enjoy your next scheduled meal is select a container from the fridge and pop it in the microwave. Further, quick and easy snacks may be stored individually as well in ziplock sandwich bags for ultra convenience. I also recommend picking up some reusable containers for your individual meals, as they're inexpensive.

Sticking to the Diet While Dining Out

Food is, always has been, and always will be the centerpiece of our social lives. You'll find it at just about every social gathering from formal to informal. The attendance at any decent restaurant on a Friday night validates that eating and food are indeed America's favorite pastimes. Unfortunately, when dieting, most individuals feel as though they're unable to enjoy or participate in the social pastime of dining out. This couldn't be further from the truth. You can easily stick to the parameters of the Cheat to Lose Diet when eating out; you'll simply have to keep a few basics in mind.

1. **Stick to Cheat to Lose portions.** Just because your entree contains two portions of protein and two portions of higher-GI/GL carbs doesn't mean that you have to eat everything on your plate. Eat one of each and bring the rest home for a quick and easy reheatable meal the next day. The portion prescription for the meal you're eating is what determines how much you should eat, whether you're at home or dining out.

2. **Order from specialty health menus when possible.** Most restaurants have a section of their menu that specifically caters to dieters. Usually this section will include both low-carb and low-fat menu options. Generally, regular entrees are loaded with hidden fat (even if they sound healthy), so the low-fat choices will contain a more normal amount of the macronutrient. Also, ordering from the low-carb menu is a smart move for low-carb days.

3. **Add, subtract, and substitute where possible.** If you're not ordering from a specialty menu, you generally have the liberty to substitute side items for a healthier choice and/or subtract an off-limits part of the meal. Depending on the day, do without the bun or roll, request whole-wheat over white, and/or substitute broccoli or other green veggies for high-fat and high-carb sides.

4. **Skip the appetizers and desserts.** Your entree should cover your protein, carbs, and/or fat needs, and most will leave you with extra to boot, so there's no need to add more via appetizers and desserts. Still, it may be difficult to just sit while others partake of an appetizer, so make the healthier choice and order a small green salad with light dressing.

By keeping the above basic guidelines in mind, you'll never have to turn down an invitation to grab a bite to eat or feel as though you're stuck at home. Be social, have fun, and enjoy life and time with those you love—all while being healthy. It can be done, and much more easily than most think.

Fast Food

A hot meal in minutes and at an economical price? There's no getting around the convenience of fast food. Unfortunately, if you're looking to improve your health through weight loss, the typical fast-food establishment provides very few, if any, options to suit your needs. In the mood for a Whopper with cheese? That'll cost you 800 calories and 50 grams of fat. Even the average 4-ounce cheeseburger totals more than 500 calories and over 25 grams of fat—and that's just the sandwich. "Value meal" it with fries and a cola and you're easily tipping over 1,000 calories. With numbers like those, it's no wonder fast-food-loving America is overweight.

And the health and obesity issues exacerbated by America's chronic ingestion of burgers and the like do not stop with the high calorie content. Ground beef patties are served on highly processed white bread, and the beef used at most establishments has a less-than-desirable fat composition. French fries are extremely high on the glycemic index and often loaded with the most unhealthful type of fat, trans fat. Sugar-laden, insulin-spiking fountain sodas and other beverages further worsen the situation, as they contain one of the most lipolytic (fat-storage-causing) sugars around—high-fructose corn syrup.

All these combinations are fat-promoting and health-demoting—results that couldn't be more in opposition to the desired outcomes of the Cheat to Lose Diet.

Now, that's not to say that all burgers are evil, but it's highly unlikely that you'll find a patty made from extremely lean, omega-3-rich, grass-fed beef at your typical fast-food joint. Luckily, there is one particular quick-service establishment that is atypical, and I'm happy to recommend Chick-fil-A as my number one choice for a hot, convenient, and *nutritious* meal on the go. From their impeccable customer service to their wide variety of healthy, nutritious menu options, Chick-fil-A is a standout among quick-service restaurants. Unlike other fast-food establishments centered around the burger, Chick-fil-A specializes in the healthier, leaner chicken breast, not the dubious "formed" patties you've become accustomed to at other institutions. Chick-fil-A serves real, 100 percent chicken breast containing the highest-quality protein, just like the kind you buy from your local grocery store.

Within Chick-fil-A's menu, there are numerous items that can be successfully incorporated into various days of the Cheat to Lose Diet; I've listed them below.

- **Cool Wraps** consist of seasoned grilled chicken breast, greens, and various vegetables (such as shredded carrots and sliced tomatoes) along with a blend of Monterey Jack and Cheddar cheeses tightly rolled in a tortilla. They are available in chargrilled, spicy, and Caesar varieties and are served with choice of dressing. *These are best consumed on higher-GI/GL days. Also be sure to ask for a low-fat or light dressing.*
- **Chargrilled Salads** consist of grilled chicken served over a bed of romaine and iceberg lettuces along with shredded carrots, red cabbage, tomatoes, and a blend of Monterey Jack and Cheddar cheeses. They are available in char-grilled and spicy/Southwest varieties. *The char-grilled variety can be consumed on any day of the diet. Just be sure your dressing choice corresponds with the day.*

The Southwest variety is best consumed on either low-GI/GL or higher-GI/GL days. Again, choose a low-fat or light dressing.

- **The Chargrilled Chicken Sandwich** is a marinated boneless breast of grilled chicken served on a toasted whole-wheat bun with dill pickle chips, green leaf lettuce, and sliced tomato. *This sandwich with its wheat bun is best consumed on either low-GI/GL or higher-GI/GL days. Enjoy without the bun on any day.*

- **Hearty Breast of Chicken Soup** consists of chunks of chicken breast, chopped carrots, and chopped celery with egg noodles in broth. *Enjoy on higher-GI/GL days.*

- **The Fresh Fruit Cup,** a mix of mandarin oranges, strawberries, red and green apples, and red grapes, is a great-tasting, nutritious alternative to the standard fried side items of fast-food restaurants. *Enjoy on either lower-GI/GL or higher-GI/GL days.*

- **The Chargrilled Chicken Sandwich Value Meal** is a great, healthy complete meal alternative to the fat-laden, highly processed value meals of other establishments if you swap the fries for a Fresh Fruit Cup and make the soda diet. *Enjoy as a main meal on low-GI/GL or higher-GI/GL days.*

- **Chick-fil-A Waffle Potato Fries and Old-Fashioned Hand-Spun Milk Shakes** should be saved for your Cheat Day (but Chick-fil-A's fries and milk shakes are some of the most delicious around).

Now, certainly Chick-fil-A is not the only fast-food restaurant with menu items acceptable to eat on the Cheat to Lose Diet—it just happens to have more than most. Still, when dining at other establishments, you can still make healthier selections by choosing the smaller burgers offered, sans the white-bread bun, and by opting for grilled over fried when it comes to other protein sources. Also, most establishments do offer at least one salad, but be careful to avoid high-calorie dressings and anything not on the approved food lists.

Tips for Staying Motivated

Establish Clear, Realistic Goals

How will you reach a goal if you don't first clearly establish one? I am continually amazed to see how many individuals begin a fitness or nutrition program with no real goal in mind. Goals such as "I want to get in better shape" or "I want to be thinner" are unacceptable—they're too ambiguous. If you want to set yourself up for success, you need to give yourself something quantifiable to shoot for. "I want to lose 20 pounds" is a good goal; "I want to lose 20 pounds in ten weeks" is even better. At the same time, make sure your goals are realistic and achievable. If you set an unrealistic goal, it's easy to become discouraged when you realize you won't be able to reach it in time. Instead, choose something that is doable while still being challenging. And once you've met the goal, reevaluate and set a new goal to achieve even more.

Review Your Goals Daily

Once you've set a clear, realistic goal, write that goal down and place it where you'll see it on a daily basis—on your bathroom mirror, your desk or PC, or even the dashboard of your car. This will constantly remind you of the mission you are on and serve as a means of accountability, as your goal is a promise to yourself.

Work with the End in Mind

See the big picture and realize that Rome wasn't built in a day. Sure, it's a cliché, but it bears repeating. The progress that you make each week is what is getting you to your ultimate goal. You may be someone who has quite a way to go, but each and every week you're looking and feeling better, and so long as you keep up the great work, before you know it you'll be right where you want to be.

Recognize the Power of Positive Self-Talk

Go back to the goals you set for yourself and make the following change: replace the word *want* with *will*. Now read your goal again. It's empowering, isn't it? Encourage yourself with positive words: *I can do it. I will achieve my goals. I will be prepared. I will not abandon the plan.* These phrases are full of power. Believe them, speak them, and watch and see how much more motivated you become.

Visualize

Another way to stay motivated is through visualization. Close your eyes and envision what it will be like and how it will feel when you reach your goals. That feeling is not far away if you continue to work hard to make your vision a reality.

Other Quick Tips for Staying on Track

Cook Meats Ahead of Time

While cooking ahead of time was discussed in general, it warrants repeating with regard to meats. Cooking protein sources in bulk at the beginning of the week will make things incredibly easy for you. Start each week by cooking up a large amount of each of your favorite protein sources. For me, this means taking time each weekend to cook several days' worth of chicken breasts, extra-lean ground beef, and fish—these are the staple protein sources I consume each week, and having them ready to go makes eating these favorites easy. (*Note:* If cooking fish ahead of time, be sure to con-

sume it within forty-eight hours of cooking, as it has a shorter refrigerator life than other meats.)

Shake a Shake for Convenience

While there's nothing quite as tasty as the nutrition shake recipes
included in Part III of the book (flavors include cookies and cream,
chocolate peanut butter, and blueberry cheesecake, just to name a
few), these recipes require the use of a blender. Unfortunately, you
won't always have the time or the luxury to use a blender when
making nutrition shakes, and this is where a shaker cup comes in
handy. Shaker cups allow you to easily mix protein powder and
water or milk and then consume the prepared shake right from
the cup. They can be purchased online for a few bucks apiece (simply type "shaker cup" in any online search engine) or at your local
nutritional supplement store. I recommend buying several and
keeping one at home and one at work.

Check Labels for Hidden Carbs, Sugars, and Calories

If you are unsure of how much to consume of a particular food or
if it's even a good food to consume, check the Nutrition Facts
label. Many products have hidden sugars and calories and should
be avoided. For example, a typical 8-ounce yogurt can easily contain more than 200 calories and over 40 grams of sugar, while the
same serving of nonfat light yogurt will provide substantially less
than half those numbers. Also, on low-carb days, be on the look-
out for hidden carbs (don't worry about fiber) in foods you may
not realize contain them. How do you know if a product contains
substantial carbs? Again, if you're unsure, it's always best to take a
few seconds and check the label.

Befriend Fruit

Not only is fruit one of the healthiest carb sources around, providing an array of nutrients, it's also the quickest and most convenient, requiring no prep time in most cases. To take full advantage of this wonder-carb source, always have a generous amount of various fruits around and reach for them often.

Always Have a Backup

As you plan your weekly menus, always have a plan B in place. Keeping a few bars or other convenient snacks handy for use in emergency-type situations shows smarts and foresight.

Use Water to Your Advantage

As simple as it might sound, downing a large glass of water is a great way to curb appetite when facing a craving. Consuming adequate water daily will also help stabilize water balance (thus reducing bloating and water retention) and promote hydration. I recommend keeping a water bottle handy and drinking enough so that you need to refill it several times throughout the day.

Cheat to Lose Daily Menus

n Part II of the book, you will be provided with sample daily menus for the Priming Phase (all three weeks), Core Phase (six weeks' worth), and Maintenance Phase (three weeks' worth) for your benefit and convenience. As you browse through this section, please keep the following in close mind:

- **Daily menus are guides.** Although you can follow them to the letter if you wish, doing so would require more time and effort than is realistic for most people, not to mention that we all differ in our likes and dislikes when it comes to the food we eat. I realize this and have included them not as absolutes, but rather to give you a wide variety of options to choose from. Within them, you should find many meals that suit your liking and which you'll want to eat more frequently.

- **The use of Metabolic Drive products is a recommendation.** Throughout the menu plans and recipes you will see that I include Metabolic Drive bars and shakes. Obviously, Metabolic Drive products are not the only meal replacement products acceptable for use with the Cheat to Lose Diet; however, I am recommending them because it is unlikely that you will find such a high-quality, great-tasting product elsewhere for a similar price. (Rest assured, I do not own any Metabolic Drive stock nor do I have any ulterior motive in recommending it.) That said, if you would like to use another meal replacement or protein powder, it's more than fine. Just be sure the product is a milk protein blend containing both whey and casein. If possible, avoid whey concentrate in favor of whey isolate and shoot for a blend containing micellar casein as the casein source. Again, it must be a blend, not a strictly whey product (whey is very quickly digested and produces an undesirable rise in insulin when consumed alone). Additionally, other meal replacement bars are not recommended for regular consumption, as the protein content of most is generally not high enough and/or the sugar content is too high and/or the protein quality is poor and/or the soy content is too high. Finally, it is not necessary that you use meal replacement products to experience success on this program; just realize that consuming strictly whole food will require a bit more planning and preparation.
- **Simple and plain is more than acceptable.** While many delicious recipes have been provided to give you plenty of options to spice up diet days, you may be someone who enjoys things on the simpler side most of the time. If so, keep in mind that meals can be as extravagant or as plain as you like so long as you follow the very

general guidelines for the type of day and meal. In chapter 6, I provided you with a wide variety of acceptable protein, fat, low-GI/GL carb, and higher-GI/GL carb sources. The most basic meals can be created by simply choosing foods from these lists. For example, meals on higher-GI/GL days call for one portion of lean protein and one portion of higher-GI/GL carbs. To easily create your own higher-GI/GL meal, first choose a lean protein source (such as chicken breast) and then choose a higher-GI/GL carb source (for example, rice). Voilà—you're done.

- **Snacks can be meals.** Simply because something is labeled as a snack doesn't mean it can only be consumed as a snack. You may consume approved protein shakes, parfaits, protein cookies, and so on—things that are typically listed as snacks on the templates—as main meals on various days if need be or if you prefer. Some days you may be busy or you may not feel like cooking, and other times you might find yourself in the mood for a specific snack when mealtime rolls around. Whatever the case, if it makes things easier, more convenient, or more enjoyable, it's the way to go.

- **Breakfast can be dinner.** Just as snacks can be meals, breakfast can be dinner. Simply because a recipe is listed as a breakfast doesn't mean it can only be consumed in the morning. The same goes for lunches and dinners. If you're in the mood for Pumpkin Pancakes for dinner, by all means go right ahead. If the stuffed peppers you prepared for dinner catch your eye in the morning, don't hesitate. Omelet for lunch? If that's what you're in the mood for, go for it. Flexibility is key to dieting success, and there is certainly plenty built into this program.

- **Whole food is important.** While nutrition shakes and the like are great for convenience, nothing compares to the fiber, phytochemical, vitamin, and mineral content of whole foods. Strive to consume at minimum two whole-food meals per day, with three or more being closer to ideal.

- **"Free" vegetables are *still* free.** Vegetables from the "free" veggies list can be added to any meal. In fact, these vegetables can be consumed at any time as an unofficial snack to fight cravings or to up your daily fiber content.

- **Salad makes a fabulous addition to any meal.** (Just make sure to season it with very-low-calorie dressing.) Also, keep in mind that a quick low-carb meal can be whipped together by adding an already prepared, refrigerated protein source (such as grilled chicken) to a large bowl of greens. Drizzle with olive oil and balsamic vinegar and you have a delicious, nutritious meal in minutes.

- **Omega-3s are essential.** Even if you're regularly consuming fish, you're probably still not getting optimal amounts of omega-3 fats from your diet alone. The simple solution: supplement. If you paid attention in chapter 3, you're well aware that this essential fatty acid possesses more health benefits than we have fingers *and* toes to count. Pick up a few bottles locally or online and supplement meals that fall a tad short on fat content.

- **Fiber is extremely important to digestive health.** Fiber can easily be added to meals by piling on the green vegetables or including a green leafy salad, or to shakes with a fiber supplement such as Metamucil. Daily intake should be in the 30- to 50-gram range for most individuals.

Priming Phase
Sample Menus

Day 1: Low Carb

Breakfast	African Bobotie (page 186)
Snack	Chocolate Peanut Butter Protein Smoothie (page 252)
Lunch	Grilled Tuna Salad (page 210)
Snack	Sliced fresh ham, mixed nuts
Dinner	Grilled salmon, mixed greens

Day 2: Low Carb

Breakfast	Tomato-Basil Omelet (page 192)
Snack	2 hard-boiled eggs, celery
Lunch	Bunless 95% lean cheeseburger, broccoli
Snack	Metabolic Drive Low-Carb Vanilla Protein Shake, 1 ounce Cheddar cheese
Dinner	Insalata Mista with Lemon-Garlic Chicken (page 230)

Day 3: Low Carb

Breakfast	Spinach and provolone omelet (1 to 2 whole eggs, plus additional whites)
Snack	Sliced grilled chicken breast, celery, all-natural peanut butter
Lunch	Pork and Vegetable Stir-Fry (page 208)
Snack	Chocolate Mint Protein Smoothie (page 252)
Dinner	Haddock with Citrus-Chili Rub (page 233), mixed greens

Day 4: Low Carb

Breakfast	Mushroom and Swiss omelet (1 to 2 whole eggs, plus additional whites)
Snack	Canned tuna mixed with relish and ⅔ to 1 tablespoon olive oil
Lunch	Filet of Sole with Black Olives and Feta Cheese (page 208)
Snack	Metabolic Drive Low-Carb Strawberry Protein Shake, 1 ounce Cheddar cheese
Dinner	Chicken with Arugula and Lemon Sauce (page 229)

Day 5: Low Carb

Breakfast	Smoked Salmon Frittata (page 191)
Snack	Café Mocha Protein Smoothie (page 253)
Lunch	Turkey breast, bacon, and Cheddar melt on low-carb tortilla
Snack	Beef jerky, mixed nuts
Dinner	Sun-Dried Tomato Pesto Chicken (page 232), mixed greens

Day 6: Low Carb

Breakfast	Spinach Scrambled Eggs with Shrimp (page 188)
Snack	Metabolic Drive Low-Carb Milk Chocolate Protein Shake, 1 ounce Cheddar cheese
Lunch	Smoked Salmon with Dill Yogurt (page 212)
Snack	Sliced flank steak, celery
Dinner	Low-Carb Chicken Fajitas (page 228)

Day 7: Low Carb

Breakfast	Scallops with eggs (1 to 2 whole eggs, plus additional whites)
Snack	Pistachio Mint Protein Smoothie (page 253)
Lunch	Sliced Sirloin with Arugula and Feta Cheese (page 209)
Snack	Canned tuna mixed with relish and ⅔ to 1 tablespoon olive oil
Dinner	Beer Can Chicken (page 228), asparagus

Day 8: Low GI/GL

Breakfast	Raw Oatmeal with Dried Fruit (page 196)
Snack	Berry Blast Protein Smoothie (page 254)
Lunch	Ground turkey and lentil soup, navel orange
Snack	Strawberry Parfait (page 266)
Dinner	Asparagus-Stuffed Chicken (page 236)

Day 9: Low GI/GL

Breakfast	Ham and egg white omelet (1 to 2 whole eggs, plus additional whites), oatmeal (plain rolled oats) topped with ground flaxseeds and strawberries
Snack	Metabolic Drive Protein Energy Bar
Lunch	Balsamic Chicken with Chickpea Puree (page 213)
Snack	Chocolate Peanut Butter Protein Cookies (page 265)
Dinner	Grilled Lamb and Couscous Salad (page 240)

Day 10: Low GI/GL

Breakfast	Fruit Crumble (page 193)
Snack	Protein Pudding (page 268)
Lunch	Chicken with Roasted Onion and Mango Salad (page 214)
Snack	Metabolic Drive Protein Energy Bar
Dinner	Lean pork chop, sweet potato, lima beans

Day 11: Low GI/GL

Breakfast	Tomato and cheese omelet (1 to 2 whole eggs, plus additional whites), navel orange
Snack	Raspberry Parfait (page 266)
Lunch	Honey-Mustard Chicken Salad (page 215)
Snack	Piña Colada Protein Smoothie (page 258)
Dinner	Zucchini Parmigiana (page 242)

Day 12: Low GI/GL

Breakfast	Breakfast Yogurt (page 192)
Snack	Blueberry Parfait (page 266)
Lunch	Smoked turkey breast and cheese on 100% whole-wheat bread, honeydew
Snack	Cinnamon Bun Protein Smoothie (page 255)
Dinner	Shepherd's Pie (page 238)

Day 13: Low GI/GL

Breakfast	Scrambled eggs (1 to 2 whole eggs, plus additional whites), black beans, strawberries
Snack	Blueberry Cheesecake Protein Smoothie (page 259)
Lunch	Warm Turkey Calzone (page 216)
Snack	Sliced fresh ham, kiwi, mixed nuts
Dinner	Grilled Lean Pork with Peach-Mango Salsa (page 238), mixed greens

Day 14: Low GI/GL

Breakfast	Stuffed French Toast (page 195)
Snack	Metabolic Drive Complete Milk Chocolate Protein Shake with skim milk
Lunch	Hamburger with Bean Puree (page 217)
Snack	Metabolic Drive Protein Energy Bar
Dinner	Grilled chicken breast, fruit salad, green beans

Day 15: Higher GI/GL

Breakfast	Apple-Carrot Muffins (page 199)
Snack	Peach Cobbler Parfait (page 267)
Lunch	Chicken noodle soup
Snack	Metabolic Drive Protein Energy Bar
Dinner	Breaded Chicken with Rice (page 243), spinach

Day 16: Higher GI/GL

Breakfast	Lumberjack's Breakfast (page 200)
Snack	Protein Pudding (page 268)
Lunch	Filet of sole, rigatoni with low-fat tomato sauce
Snack	Strawberry Parfait (page 266)
Dinner	Green Pea Mashed Potatoes with Minced Beef (page 243)

Day 17: Higher GI/GL

Breakfast	Chocolate Protein-Packed Cheerios (page 198)
Snack	Metabolic Drive Protein Energy Bar
Lunch	Asian Chicken Wraps (page 219)
Snack	Chocolate-Banana Protein Smoothie (page 258)
Dinner	Turkey Burger with Mixed Berry Sauce (page 248), mixed green salad with light low-calorie dressing

Day 18: Higher GI/GL

Breakfast	Pumpkin Pancakes (page 201)
Snack	Blueberry Parfait (page 266)
Lunch	Oven-Roasted Chicken Breast with Roasted Pear Sandwich (page 223)
Snack	S'mores Protein Smoothie (page 260)
Dinner	Salmon, fettuccine with low-fat Alfredo sauce, green beans

Day 19: Higher GI/GL

Breakfast	Banana Breakfast Sandwich (page 198)
Snack	Metabolic Drive Complete Vanilla Protein Shake
Lunch	BBQ Chicken Sandwich (page 222)
Snack	Metabolic Drive Protein Energy Bar
Dinner	Grilled Chicken Breast, spaghetti with low-fat tomato sauce, mixed green salad with light low-calorie dressing

Day 20: Higher GI/GL

Breakfast	100% whole-wheat English muffin with grape jelly, nonfat cottage cheese
Snack	Chocolate Lover's Protein Smoothie (page 260)
Lunch	Rotis (page 224)
Snack	Peaches and Cream Protein Smoothie (page 255)
Dinner	Turkey Pizza (page 245)

Day 21: Cheat Day

Work with Your Body, Not Against It!

Core Phase
Sample Menus

Day 1: Low Carb

Breakfast	Feta Cheese and Leek Omelet (page 187)
Snack	Sliced grilled chicken breast, mixed nuts
Lunch	Roast beef, lettuce, and tomato on low-carb tortilla
Snack	Metabolic Drive Low-Carb Strawberry Protein Shake, 1 ounce Cheddar cheese
Dinner	Satay Chicken with Spicy Peanut Sauce (page 234), asparagus

Day 2: Low Carb

Breakfast	Scrambled egg whites, bacon
Snack	Metabolic Drive Low-Carb Strawberry Protein Shake, 1 ounce Cheddar cheese
Lunch	Swordfish with Steamed Green Beans (page 212)
Snack	Beef jerky, mixed nuts
Dinner	Spicy Chicken and Roasted Pepper Salad (page 235)

Day 3: Low GI/GL

Breakfast	Breakfast Parfait (page 195)
Snack	Metabolic Drive Protein Energy Bar
Lunch	Chicken Caesar Pita (page 217)
Snack	Peaches and Cream Protein Smoothie (page 255)
Dinner	95% lean ground beef and bean chili (no rice)

Day 4: Low GI/GL

Breakfast	Metabolic Drive Protein Energy Bar, apple
Snack	Vanilla Protein Cookies (page 265)
Lunch	Tuna Steak with Olive Pesto (page 218)
Snack	Blueberry Parfait (page 266)
Dinner	Lean roast beef with lettuce and tomato on 100% whole-wheat bread, pear

Day 5: Higher GI/GL

Breakfast	Turkey Sausage Crepes (page 205)
Snack	Metabolic Drive Protein Energy Bar
Lunch	Chicken Cacciatore Wraps (page 220)
Snack	Banana-Coconut Protein Smoothie (page 259)
Dinner	Smoked salmon with whole-grain rice, snow peas

Day 6: Higher GI/GL

Breakfast	Chocolate Protein-Packed Cheerios (page 198)
Snack	Vanilla Protein Cookies (page 265)
Lunch	Grilled chicken breast, rigatoni with low-fat tomato sauce
Snack	Metabolic Drive Complete Milk Chocolate Protein Shake with skim milk
Dinner	Filet of sole, whole-grain rice

Day 7: Cheat Day

Work with Your Body, Not Against It!

Day 8: Low Carb

Breakfast	African Bobotie (page 186)
Snack	Chocolate Peanut Butter Protein Smoothie (page 252)
Lunch	Grilled Tuna Salad (page 210)
Snack	Sliced fresh ham, mixed nuts
Dinner	Grilled salmon, mixed greens

Day 9: Low Carb

Breakfast	Low-carb breakfast burrito
Snack	Metabolic Drive Low-Carb Vanilla Protein Shake, 1 ounce Cheddar cheese
Lunch	Sliced lean pork roast, mixed greens
Snack	Hard-boiled eggs, celery
Dinner	Smoked Salmon with Portobello Mushrooms and Asparagus (page 231)

Day 10: Low GI/GL

Breakfast	Whole-Wheat Pancakes (page 197), **Metabolic Drive Low-Carb Strawberry Protein Shake**
Snack	Chocolate Peanut Butter Protein Cookies (page 265)
Lunch	**Grilled chicken breast, fruit salad**
Snack	Peach Cobbler Parfait (page 267)
Dinner	Lamb Chops with Beet-and-Orange Salad (page 241)

Day 11: Low GI/GL

Breakfast	Stuffed French Toast (page 195)
Snack	**Metabolic Drive Complete Milk Chocolate Protein Shake with skim milk**
Lunch	Hamburger with Bean Puree (page 217)
Snack	**Metabolic Drive Protein Energy Bar**
Dinner	**Grilled chicken breast, green beans, fruit salad**

Day 12: Higher GI/GL

Breakfast	Banana-Yogurt Waffles (page 202)
Snack	**Metabolic Drive Protein Energy Bar**
Lunch	Oven-Roasted Turkey and Cucumber Sandwich (page 221)
Snack	Apple-Cinnamon Oblivion Protein Smoothie (page 254)
Dinner	**Grilled chicken breast, whole-grain rice, greens**

Day 13: Higher GI/GL

Breakfast	Apple-Carrot Muffins (page 199)
Snack	Peach Cobbler Parfait (page 267)
Lunch	Chicken noodle soup
Snack	Metabolic Drive Protein Energy Bar
Dinner	Steak with Spicy Chili Cream and White Rice (page 244), **green beans**

Day 14: Cheat Day

Work with Your Body, Not Against It!

Day 15: Low Carb

Breakfast	Spinach and provolone omelet (1 to 2 whole eggs, plus additional whites)
Snack	Sliced grilled chicken breast, celery, all-natural peanut butter
Lunch	Pork and Vegetable Stir-Fry (page 208)
Snack	Chocolate Mint Protein Smoothie (page 252)
Dinner	Haddock with Citrus-Chili Rub (page 233), **mixed greens**

Day 16: Low Carb

Breakfast	Salmon and Dill Omelet (page 190)
Snack	Beef jerky, mixed nuts
Lunch	Spicy Chili-Rubbed Salmon with Grilled Zucchini (page 210), mixed greens with light low-calorie dressing
Snack	Metabolic Drive Low-Carb Milk Chocolate Protein Shake, 1 ounce Cheddar cheese
Dinner	Flank steak, mixed greens

Day 17: Low GI/GL

Breakfast	Tomato and cheese omelet (1 to 2 whole eggs, plus additional whites), navel orange
Snack	Raspberry Parfait (page 266)
Lunch	Honey-Mustard Chicken Salad (page 215)
Snack	Piña Colada Protein Smoothie (page 258)
Dinner	Zucchini Parmigiana (page 242)

Day 18: Low GI/GL

Breakfast	Breakfast Yogurt (page 192)
Snack	Blueberry Parfait (page 266)
Lunch	Smoked turkey breast and Swiss cheese on 100% whole-wheat bread, honeydew
Snack	Cinnamon Bun Protein Smoothie (page 255)
Dinner	Shepherd's Pie (page 238)

Day 19: Higher GI/GL

Breakfast	Ham steak with 100% whole-wheat toast
Snack	Strawberry-Banana Protein Smoothie (page 257)
Lunch	Salmon with whole-grain rice
Snack	Blueberry Parfait (page 266)
Dinner	Chicken Potpie (page 246)

Day 20: Higher GI/GL

Breakfast	Roasted Potato Cheese Pie (page 204)
Snack	Key Lime Pie Protein Smoothie (page 257)
Lunch	Sirloin Steak with Peach-Cucumber Salsa and Grilled Red Potatoes (page 221)
Snack	Metabolic Drive Protein Energy Bar
Dinner	Grilled chicken breast, spaghetti with low-fat tomato sauce, mixed green salad with light low-calorie dressing

Day 21: Cheat Day

Work with Your Body, Not Against It!

Day 22: Low Carb

Breakfast	Chicken Sausage Frittata (page 189)
Snack	Hard-boiled eggs, celery
Lunch	Bunless 95% lean cheeseburger with broccoli
Snack	Metabolic Drive Low-Carb Vanilla Protein Shake, 1 ounce Cheddar cheese
Dinner	Insalata Mista with Lemon-Garlic Chicken (page 230)

Day 23: Low carb

Breakfast	Scallops with eggs (1 to 2 whole eggs, plus additional whites)
Snack	Pistachio Mint Protein Smoothie (page 253)
Lunch	Sliced Sirloin with Arugula and Feta Cheese (page 209)
Snack	Canned tuna mixed with relish and ⅔ to 1 tablespoon olive oil
Dinner	Beer Can Chicken (page 228), asparagus

Day 24: Low GI/GL

Breakfast	Breakfast Granola (page 194)
Snack	Berry Blast Protein Smoothie (page 254)
Lunch	Ground turkey and lentil soup, navel orange
Snack	Strawberry Parfait (page 266)
Dinner	Asparagus-Stuffed Chicken (page 236)

Breakfast	Egg and cheese omelet (1 to 2 whole eggs, plus additional whites), oatmeal (plain rolled oats) topped with strawberries
Snack	Chocolate Peanut Butter Protein Cookies (page 265)
Lunch	Grilled salmon with lima beans, navel orange
Snack	Creamy Strawberry Passion Protein Smoothie (page 256)
Dinner	Caramelized Onions and Pork Chops (page 237), broccoli

Day 26: Higher GI/GL

Breakfast	Protein Polenta with Bananas and Maple Syrup (page 203)
Snack	Protein Pudding (page 268)
Lunch	Filet of sole, rigatoni with low-fat tomato sauce
Snack	Strawberry Parfait (page 266)
Dinner	Sloppy Joes on 100% Whole-Wheat Buns (page 245)

Day 27: Higher GI/GL

Breakfast	Fresh ham and egg-white sandwich on 100% whole-wheat English muffin
Snack	Metabolic Drive Protein Energy Bar

Lunch	Salmon with whole-grain rice and green beans
Snack	Oats and Honey Protein Smoothie (page 256)
Dinner	Turkey Sausage with Potato Cakes (page 249)

Day 28: Cheat Day

Work with Your Body, Not Against It!

Day 29: Low Carb

Breakfast	Smoked Salmon Frittata (page 191)
Snack	Café Mocha Protein Smoothie (page 253)
Lunch	Turkey breast, bacon, and Cheddar melt on low-carb tortilla
Snack	Beef jerky, mixed nuts
Dinner	Sun-Dried Tomato Pesto Chicken (page 232), mixed greens

Day 30: Low Carb

| Breakfast | Smoked Chipotle Cheese Omelet (page 187) |
| Snack | Metabolic Drive Low-Carb Milk Chocolate Protein Shake, 1 ounce Cheddar cheese |

Lunch	Salmon Kebabs and Green Beans (page 211)
Snack	Canned tuna mixed with relish and ⅔ to 1 tablespoon olive oil
Dinner	New York strip steak (trim fat), steamed broccoli

Day 31: Low GI/GL

Breakfast	Strawberry Parfait (page 266), **fresh cherries**
Snack	Oats and Honey Protein Smoothie (page 256)
Lunch	Hawaiian Baked Beans (page 220)
Snack	**Sliced flank steak, pear**
Dinner	Bell Peppers Stuffed with Chicken and Whole-Grain Rice (page 239)

Day 32: Low GI/GL

Breakfast	Fruit Crumble (page 193)
Snack	Protein Pudding (page 268)
Lunch	Chicken with Roasted Onion and Mango Salad (page 214)
Snack	**Metabolic Drive Protein Energy Bar**
Dinner	**Lean pork chop, sweet potato, lima beans**

Day 33: Higher GI/GL

Breakfast	Chocolate Protein-Packed Cheerios (page 198)
Snack	Cookies and Cream Protein Smoothie (page 261)

Lunch	Sliced grilled chicken breast on 100% whole-wheat toast
Snack	Strawberry Parfait (page 266)
Dinner	Grilled tiger shrimp, bow-tie pasta with low-fat tomato sauce

Day 34: Higher GI/GL

Breakfast	Turkey Polenta Cakes (page 202)
Snack	Metabolic Drive Protein Energy Bar
Lunch	Asian Chicken Wraps (page 219)
Snack	Chocolate-Banana Protein Smoothie (page 258)
Dinner	Turkey Burger with Mixed Berry Sauce (page 248), mixed green salad with light low-calorie dressing

Day 35: Cheat Day

Work with Your Body,
Not Against It!

Day 36: Low Carb

Breakfast	Mushroom and Swiss omelet (1 to 2 whole eggs, plus additional whites)

Snack	Canned salmon mixed with relish and ⅔ to 1 tablespoon olive oil
Lunch	Filet of Sole with Black Olives and Feta Cheese (page 208)
Snack	Metabolic Drive Low-Carb Strawberry Protein Shake, 1 ounce Cheddar cheese
Dinner	Chicken with Arugula and Lemon Sauce (page 229)

Day 37: Low Carb

Breakfast	Spinach Scrambled Eggs with Shrimp (page 188)
Snack	Metabolic Drive Low-Carb Milk Chocolate Protein Shake, 1 ounce Cheddar cheese
Lunch	Smoked Salmon with Dill Yogurt (page 212)
Snack	Sliced flank steak, celery
Dinner	Low-Carb Chicken Fajitas (page 228)

Day 38: Low GI/GL

Breakfast	Ham and egg-white omelet, oatmeal (plain rolled oats) topped with ground flaxseeds and strawberries
Snack	Metabolic Drive Protein Energy Bar
Lunch	Balsamic Chicken with Chickpea Puree (page 213)
Snack	Chocolate Peanut Butter Protein Cookies (page 265)
Dinner	Grilled Lamb and Couscous Salad (page 234)

Day 39: Low GI/GL

Breakfast	Scrambled eggs (1 to 2 whole eggs, plus additional whites), refried beans, strawberries
Snack	Blueberry Cheesecake Protein Smoothie (page 259)
Lunch	Warm Turkey Calzone (page 216)
Snack	Sliced fresh ham, apple, mixed nuts
Dinner	Grilled Lean Pork with Peach-Mango Salsa (page 238), mixed greens

Day 40: Higher GI/GL

Breakfast	Pumpkin Pancakes (page 201)
Snack	Blueberry Parfait (page 266)
Lunch	Sun-Dried Tomato Pesto Pizza (page 225)
Snack	S'mores Protein Smoothie (page 260)
Dinner	Salmon, fettuccine with low-fat Alfredo sauce, green beans

Day 41: Higher GI/GL

Breakfast	100% whole-wheat English muffin with grape jelly, nonfat cottage cheese
Snack	Chocolate Lover's Protein Smoothie (page 260)
Lunch	Rotis (page 224)
Snack	Peaches and Cream Protein Smoothie (page 255)
Dinner	Turkey Pizza (page 245)

Day 42: Cheat Day

Work with Your Body,
Not Against It!

Maintenance Phase Sample Menus

Note: As a reminder, per the 90 Percent Rule,
you may substitute any three meals weekly
with Cheat Meals during this phase.

Day 1: Low Carb

Breakfast	Salmon and Dill Omelet (page 190)
Snack	Beef jerky, mixed nuts
Lunch	Spicy Chili-Rubbed Salmon with Grilled Zucchini (page 210), mixed greens with light low-calorie dressing
Snack	Metabolic Drive Low-Carb Milk Chocolate Protein Shake, 1 ounce Cheddar cheese
Dinner	Flank steak, mixed greens

Day 2: Low Carb

Breakfast	Scrambled egg whites, bacon
Snack	Metabolic Drive Low-Carb Strawberry Protein Shake, 1 ounce Cheddar cheese
Lunch	Swordfish with Steamed Green Beans (page 212)
Snack	Beef jerky, mixed nuts
Dinner	Spicy Chicken and Roasted Pepper Salad (page 235)

Day 3: Low GI/GL

Breakfast	Breakfast Parfait (page 195)
Snack	Metabolic Drive Protein Energy Bar
Lunch	Chicken Caesar Pita (page 217)
Snack	Peaches and Cream Protein Smoothie (page 252)
Dinner	Cheat to Lose Easy Chili (page 236)

Day 4: Higher GI/GL

Breakfast	Banana-Yogurt Waffles (page 202)
Snack	Metabolic Drive Protein Energy Bar
Lunch	Oven-Roasted Turkey and Cucumber Sandwich (page 221)
Snack	Apple-Cinnamon Oblivion Protein Smoothie (page 254)
Dinner	Grilled chicken breast, whole-grain rice, greens

Day 5: Low GI/GL

Breakfast	Strawberry Parfait (page 266), fresh cherries
Snack	Oats and Honey Protein Smoothie (page 256)
Lunch	Hawaiian Baked Beans (page 220)
Snack	Sliced flank steak, pear
Dinner	Bell Peppers Stuffed with Chicken and Whole-Grain Rice (page 239)

Day 6: Higher GI/GL

Breakfast	Turkey Sausage Crepes (page 205)
Snack	Metabolic Drive Protein Energy Bar
Lunch	Chicken Cacciatore Wraps (page 220)
Snack	Banana-Coconut Protein Smoothie (page 259)
Dinner	Smoked salmon, whole-grain rice, snow peas

Day 7: Low GI/GL

Breakfast	Egg and cheese omelet (1 to 2 whole eggs, plus additional whites), oatmeal (plain rolled oats) topped with strawberries
Snack	Chocolate Peanut Butter Protein Cookies (page 265)
Lunch	Grilled salmon, lima beans, navel orange
Snack	Creamy Strawberry Passion Protein Smoothie (page 256)
Dinner	Caramelized Onions and Pork Chops (page 237), broccoli

Day 8: Higher GI/GL

Breakfast	Fresh ham and egg-white sandwich on 100% whole-wheat English muffin
Snack	Metabolic Drive Protein Energy Bar
Lunch	Salmon, whole-grain rice, green beans
Snack	Oats and Honey Protein Smoothie (page 256)
Dinner	Turkey Sausage with Potato Cakes (page 249)

Day 9: Low GI/GL

Breakfast	Metabolic Drive Protein Energy Bar, apple
Snack	Vanilla Protein Cookies (page 265)
Lunch	Tuna Steak with Olive Pesto (page 218)
Snack	Blueberry Parfait (page 266)
Dinner	Lean roast beef with lettuce and tomato on 100% whole-wheat bread, pear

Day 10: Higher GI/GL

Breakfast	Chocolate Protein-Packed Cheerios (page 198)
Snack	Cookies and Cream Protein Smoothie (page 261)
Lunch	Sliced grilled chicken breast on 100% whole-wheat toast
Snack	Strawberry Parfait (page 266)
Dinner	Grilled tiger shrimp, bow-tie pasta with low-fat tomato sauce

Day 11: Low GI/GL

Breakfast	Raw Oatmeal with Dried Fruit (page 196)
Snack	Berry Blast Protein Smoothie (page 254)
Lunch	Ground turkey and lentil soup, navel orange
Snack	Strawberry Parfait (page 266)
Dinner	Asparagus-Stuffed Chicken (page 236)

Day 12: Higher GI/GL

Breakfast	Apple-Carrot Muffins (page 199)
Snack	Peach Cobbler Parfait (page 266)
Lunch	Chicken noodle soup, mixed green salad with light low-calorie dressing
Snack	Metabolic Drive Protein Energy Bar
Dinner	Breaded Chicken with Rice (page 243), spinach

Day 13: Low GI/GL

Breakfast	Ham and egg-white omelet, oatmeal (plain rolled oats) topped with ground flaxseeds and strawberries
Snack	Metabolic Drive Protein Energy Bar
Lunch	Balsamic Chicken with Chickpea Puree (page 213)
Snack	Chocolate Peanut Butter Protein Cookies (page 265)
Dinner	Grilled Lamb and Couscous Salad (page 240)

Day 14: Higher GI/GL

Breakfast	100% whole-wheat English muffin with grape jelly, nonfat cottage cheese
Snack	Chocolate Lover's Protein Smoothie (page 260)
Lunch	Rotis (page 224)
Snack	Peaches and Cream Protein Smoothie (page 255)
Dinner	Turkey Pizza (page 245)

Day 15: Low GI/GL

Breakfast	Fruit Crumble (page 193)
Snack	Protein Pudding (page 268)
Lunch	Chicken with Roasted Onion and Mango Salad (page 214)
Snack	Metabolic Drive Protein Energy Bar
Dinner	Lean pork chop, sweet potato, lima beans

Day 16: Higher GI/GL

Breakfast	Chocolate Protein-Packed Cheerios (page 198)
Snack	Metabolic Drive Protein Energy Bar
Lunch	Asian Chicken Wraps (page 219)
Snack	Chocolate-Banana Protein Smoothie (page 258)
Dinner	Turkey Burger with Mixed Berry Sauce (page 248), mixed green salad with light low-calorie dressing

Day 17: Low GI/GL

Breakfast	Tomato and cheese omelet (1 to 2 whole eggs, plus additional whites), navel orange
Snack	Raspberry Parfait (page 266)
Lunch	Honey-Mustard Chicken Salad (page 215)
Snack	Piña Colada Protein Smoothie (page 258)
Dinner	Zucchini Parmigiana (page 242)

Day 18: Higher GI/GL

Breakfast	Lumberjack's Breakfast (page 200)
Snack	Protein Pudding (page 268)
Lunch	Filet of sole, rigatoni with low-fat tomato sauce
Snack	Strawberry Parfait (page 266)
Dinner	Green Pea Mashed Potatoes with Minced Beef (page 243)

Day 19: Low GI/GL

Breakfast	Breakfast Yogurt (page 192)
Snack	Blueberry Parfait (page 266)
Lunch	Smoked turkey breast and cheese on 100% whole-wheat bread, honeydew
Snack	Cinnamon Bun Protein Smoothie (page 255)
Dinner	Shepherd's Pie (page 238)

Day 20: Higher GI/GL

Breakfast	Pumpkin Pancakes (page 201)
Snack	Blueberry Parfait (page 266)
Lunch	Oven-Roasted Chicken Breast with Roasted Pear Sandwich (page 223)
Snack	S'mores Protein Smoothie (page 260)
Dinner	Salmon, fettuccine with low-fat Alfredo sauce, green beans

Day 21: Low GI/GL

Breakfast	Stuffed French Toast (page 195)
Snack	Metabolic Drive Complete Milk Chocolate Protein Shake with skim milk
Lunch	Hamburger with Bean Puree (page 217)
Snack	Metabolic Drive Protein Energy Bar
Dinner	Grilled chicken breast, fruit salad, green beans

PART III

Cheat to Lose Recipes

My friend and colleague Dr. John Berardi has provided recipes for seventy-five delicious breakfasts, lunches, and dinners. Additionally, I have included a number of quick and easy snack recipes, and nearly twenty of my favorite nutrition smoothie blends for ultra-convenient, great-tasting meals on the go. As you browse through this section, please keep the following in mind:

- **Recipe portions are not universal.** With recipes, exact amounts of ingredients must be given, otherwise you'd have no idea how much of what to use. Still, as mentioned in chapter 4, people of different sizes require different amounts of food—this is the reasoning behind the use of the hand/fist portion method. The recipes included in the book have been designed to yield meals sized for the average person. That said, the size of these meals may be too small or too large for you depending on your body size. When trying recipes, if the portions are too big, only eat the prescribed amount for your size and alter the recipe next time so that it will yield the appropriate portion. Remember, it is always better to underestimate than to overconsume.

- **Recipes yield multiple servings.** Most recipes yield two servings; this makes eating with a partner easy, or the additional serving can simply be saved for a later meal. Some recipes (mostly dinners) yield four servings, which will feed a family (or again, extra servings can be saved for later meals). Preparing in bulk? Double or triple the recipe. Want a single serving? Halve the recipe. The number of servings each recipe yields is located after all cooking instructions, so you're never in doubt of how many servings the listed ingredients will produce.

- **You can use canned, frozen, or fresh vegetables.** While some recipes call for fresh vegetables, frozen or canned versions may be substituted for convenience if necessary. That said, there should be no added sugars, syrups, or calories in any prepackaged product you use.

Breakfast Recipes

African Bobotie (Low Carb)

1 pound 95% lean ground beef

Cooking spray

1 onion, chopped

Grated rind and juice from 1 lemon

2 tablespoons tomato paste

1 tablespoon nonfat plain yogurt

2 tablespoons curry powder

Salt to taste

1 egg

1 cup egg whites (approximately 8 eggs)

1 tablespoon milk

Preheat the oven to 300°F. In an oven-safe skillet over medium heat, sauté the beef until browned, 10 to 12 minutes. Drain and set aside. Lightly coat the same skillet with cooking spray and sauté the onion until soft. Transfer the beef back into the skillet. Add the lemon rind and juice, tomato paste, yogurt, curry powder, and salt. Combine well, then pack down tightly, leaving an even surface. Remove the skillet from the heat.

Whisk together the egg, egg whites, and milk until thoroughly blended. Pour the egg mixture over the beef. Carefully place the skillet in the oven and bake until the eggs are golden brown, 15 to 20 minutes.

Serves 4

Feta Cheese and Leek Omelet (Low Carb)

2 small zucchini, finely chopped
2 leeks (white parts only), finely chopped
1½ tablespoons olive oil
Salt and pepper to taste
1 egg
1 cup egg whites (approximately 8 eggs)
1 tablespoon milk
Handful of fresh basil, chopped
4 ounces feta cheese, crumbled

In a nonstick skillet over medium heat, sauté the zucchini and leeks in the olive oil until lightly browned, approximately 5 minutes. Add salt and pepper. In a separate bowl, whisk together the egg, egg whites, and milk until frothy. Pour the egg mixture into the skillet, topping it off with the basil and feta cheese. Reduce the heat to low and continue cooking, occasionally lifting one side of the omelet and tipping the skillet so that any uncooked mixture will run underneath, until the eggs are fully cooked, 8 to 10 minutes.

Serves 2

Smoked Chipotle Cheese Omelet (Low Carb)

1 onion, finely diced
1 green pepper, finely diced
1 teaspoon olive oil
½ garlic clove, minced

1 egg

1 cup egg whites (approximately 8 eggs)

2 tablespoons milk

2 teaspoons smoked chipotle Tabasco sauce

Salt and pepper to taste

2 tablespoons finely chopped parsley

2 tablespoons cottage cheese

2 tablespoons shredded Cheddar cheese

1 teaspoon Parmesan cheese (optional)

In a nonstick skillet over medium heat, sauté the onion and pepper in the olive oil until lightly browned, approximately 5 minutes. Add the garlic. In a separate bowl, whisk together the egg, egg whites, milk, and Tabasco until frothy. Pour the egg mixture into the skillet, reduce the heat to low, and cover with a lid. Cook, occasionally lifting one side of the omelet and tipping the skillet so that any uncooked mixture will run underneath, until the top is fully cooked, 8 to 10 minutes. Add the salt, pepper, and parsley. Place the cheeses on one side of the omelet and gently flip the other half over to cover the cheese. Remove from heat and cover with the lid, allowing 1 to 2 minutes for the cheese to melt.

Serves 2

Spinach Scrambled Eggs with Shrimp (Low Carb)

½ cup spinach

1 egg

1 cup egg whites (approximately 8 eggs)

½ teaspoon fish sauce

1 green onion (white and green parts), finely chopped

1½ tablespoons olive oil

10 large shrimp, peeled and deveined

Fill a small pot one-quarter full with water and bring to a boil. Add the spinach and cook until soft, 30 to 60 seconds; remove from the heat and drain. Combine the spinach, egg, egg whites, and fish sauce in a blender and mix on medium speed for 30 seconds.

In a nonstick skillet over medium heat, sauté the green onion in the olive oil until lightly browned. Add the shrimp and cook for 2 minutes on each side. Pour the spinach and egg mixture over the shrimp and let everything sit untouched for 30 seconds. Scramble the eggs until fully cooked.

Serves 2

Chicken Sausage Frittata (Low Carb)

1 3-ounce chicken sausage

½ tablespoon olive oil

½ cup grated zucchini

1 garlic clove, minced

1 cup egg whites (approximately 8 eggs)

1 teaspoon Dijon mustard

5 fresh basil leaves, finely chopped

Salt to taste

Remove the sausage from its casing by slitting one end and squeezing out the meat. In a nonstick skillet over medium heat, sauté the sausage meat in the olive oil until fully cooked and gray in color, approximately 5 minutes. Add the zucchini and garlic. Whisk the egg whites in a small bowl, then add the mustard and whisk again. Pour the egg whites over the sausage mixture and sprinkle with the basil and salt. Cover the skillet and reduce the heat to low. Continue cooking for 5 minutes, occasionally lifting one side of the frittata and tipping the skillet so that any uncooked mixture will run underneath, until the frittata appears dry.

Serves 2

Salmon and Dill Omelet (Low Carb)

Cooking spray
1 cup sliced mushrooms
½ cup finely chopped onion
1 egg
1 cup egg whites (approximately 8 eggs)
¼ cup chopped flat-leaf parsley
¼ cup finely minced dill
3½ ounces smoked salmon, cut into strips
½ cup crumbled feta cheese

Lightly coat a nonstick skillet with cooking spray and place over medium heat. Sauté the mushrooms and onion until the mushrooms shrink slightly and the onion is golden. Combine the egg, egg whites, and parsley in a blender and mix on high speed for 5 seconds. Add the dill to the skillet, then pour in the eggs. Reduce the heat to low, cover, and cook, occasionally lifting one side of the omelet and tipping the skillet so that any uncooked mixture will run underneath, for 6 to 7 minutes, until the top is fully cooked. Remove the lid and lay the salmon over the eggs; top the fish with the cheese. Cover and continue cooking for an additional 3 minutes.

Serves 2

Smoked Salmon Frittata (Low Carb)

1 cup chopped asparagus
½ cup finely chopped onion
1 tablespoon olive oil
1 cup egg whites (approximately 8 eggs)
1 egg
3½ ounces smoked salmon, cut into strips
½ cup chopped basil
Salt and pepper to taste

In a nonstick skillet over medium heat, sauté the asparagus and onion in the olive oil until soft. In a separate bowl, whisk the egg and egg whites. When the vegetables have almost reached the desired tenderness, reduce the heat to low and pour in the eggs. Immediately add the salmon and basil. Cover the skillet with a lid and continue to cook on low for another 10 minutes, occasionally lifting one side of the frittata and tipping the skillet so that any uncooked mixture will run underneath, until the frittata appears dry on top. Season with salt and pepper.

Serves 2

Tomato-Basil Omelet (Low Carb)

1 tablespoon finely chopped fresh rosemary

1½ tablespoons olive oil

2 tablespoons diced canned tomatoes

1 garlic clove, minced

½ cup chopped fresh basil

1 egg

1 cup egg whites (approximately 8 eggs)

2 tablespoons tomato juice from can

Salt and pepper to taste

In a nonstick skillet over medium heat, heat the rosemary in the olive oil for 30 seconds. Add the tomatoes, garlic, and basil. Cook for approximately 3 minutes, just until the tomatoes are soft. Separately, whisk together the egg, egg whites, and tomato juice. Add the egg mixture to the skillet, cover, and cook until the top is fully cooked, occasionally lifting one edge of the omelet and tipping the skillet so that any uncooked mixture will run underneath. Season with salt and pepper.

Serves 2

Breakfast Yogurt (Low GI/GL)

2 medium peaches

1 tablespoon mint leaves

2 scoops (40 grams protein) Vanilla Metabolic Drive Low-Carb

6 ounces nonfat plain yogurt

Fill a medium pot halfway with water and bring to a boil. Submerge the peaches completely and boil for 1 to 2 minutes. Remove the peaches from the pot and let cool in a bowl for about 5 minutes or until cool enough to handle. Peel off the skin if desired. Remove the pits, cut the fruit into wedges, and place in the blender with the mint. Puree on high until smooth.

Mix the puree with the protein powder in a large bowl. Add the yogurt and mix thoroughly. Serve cold or at room temperature.

Serves 2

Fruit Crumble (Low GI/GL)

1 cup rolled oats

2 ounces unsweetened applesauce

½ teaspoon ginger

3 tablespoons freshly squeezed orange juice

1 cup fresh or frozen raspberries, thawed if frozen

2 scoops (40 grams protein) Vanilla Metabolic Drive Low-Carb

4 ounces nonfat plain yogurt

1 tablespoon true-to-measure Equal (optional)

Preheat the oven to 350°F. Blend the oats in a blender until pulverized to a flour. In a small bowl, mix the oat flour, applesauce, ginger, and orange juice to form a paste. Spread on a baking sheet lined with parchment paper. Bake for 12 minutes. When finished, the mixture should be spongy. Cool and then crumble into small, chewy bits. Set aside.

Puree the berries in a blender on low speed. Keeping the blender on, slowly add the protein powder a little at a time until well blended with the berries. If the mixture becomes too thick, add a little water (1 teaspoon to start) to make it more liquid. Divide the yogurt evenly between two bowls and top with half the berry mixture, then half the crumbles. Sprinkle with Equal if desired and serve.

Serves 2

Breakfast Granola (Low GI/GL)

½ cup rolled oats

2 scoops (40 grams protein) Vanilla Metabolic Drive Low-Carb

1 tablespoon white sesame seeds

¼ cup unsweetened coconut

2 tablespoons honey

2 tablespoons raisins

1 tablespoon sugar-free maple syrup

Nonfat plain yogurt (optional)

½ teaspoon grated lemon zest (optional)

Preheat the oven to 300°F. In a bowl, mix the oats, protein powder, sesame seeds, coconut, honey, raisins, and maple syrup. Spread on a baking sheet lined with parchment paper. Bake until the granola turns light golden brown, about 30 minutes, stirring the granola every 10 minutes. When cool, break up into chunks. Serve with a scoop of nonfat plain yogurt mixed with lemon zest, if desired.

Serves 2

Breakfast Parfait (Low GI/GL)

1 cup fresh or frozen blueberries, thawed if frozen

1 tablespoon cornstarch

2 scoops (40 grams protein) Vanilla Metabolic Drive Low-Carb

4 ounces nonfat plain yogurt

1 tablespoon true-to-measure Equal

1 cup Breakfast Granola (page 194)

Make the blueberry sauce by combining the blueberries and ½ to ¾ cup of water in a small pot. Add the cornstarch and simmer until the sauce is thick. Cool and reserve ½ cup; refrigerate the remainder for another use.

In a medium bowl, mix the protein powder with the yogurt and Equal. Spoon a little blueberry sauce into the bottom of two parfait glasses. Add a layer of granola and then a layer of yogurt. Continue layering until all the ingredients have been used up. Serve cold.

Serves 2

Stuffed French Toast (Low GI/GL)

4 ounces nonfat cottage cheese

1 scoop (20 grams protein) Vanilla Metabolic Drive Low-Carb

1 tablespoon raisins

½ cup egg whites (approximately 4 eggs)

1 teaspoon cinnamon

2 tablespoons skim milk

½ cup rolled oats

2 large slices 12-grain or 100% whole-wheat bread

1 tablespoon raspberries, strawberries, or blueberries

1 teaspoon true-to-measure Equal (optional)

In a blender, blend the cottage cheese until smooth. When finished, remove to a medium bowl and mix in the protein powder and raisins. Set aside. In another bowl, whisk together the egg whites, cinnamon, and milk. Set aside. Place the oats on a plate. Preheat a skillet over medium-high heat.

Fold each slice of bread in half to create a pocket. Fill each pocket with half the cottage cheese mixture. Dip the folded, stuffed bread into the egg mixture, then coat with the oats. Cook until golden brown, approximately 3 minutes on each side. Garnish with berries and Equal if desired.

Serves 2

Raw Oatmeal with Dried Fruit (Low GI/GL)

⅓ cup dried apricots

¼ cup raisins

⅓ cup dried mango

⅓ cup rolled oats

2 scoops (40 grams protein) Vanilla Metabolic Drive Low-Carb

½ cup nonfat plain yogurt

⅔ cup skim milk

Cut the dried fruit into small pieces. Mix the fruit with the oats and protein powder. Add the yogurt and milk and mix well.

Serves 2

Whole-Wheat Pancakes
(Low GI/GL)

¾ cup whole-wheat flour

2 teaspoons baking powder

3 tablespoons true-to-measure Equal

1 egg white

½ cup skim milk

Cooking spray

2 small handfuls of mixed berries

In a large bowl, mix the flour, baking powder, and Equal. In a separate bowl, whisk together the egg white and milk, then add to the flour along with ½ cup water. Mix just until combined.

Heat a nonstick skillet over medium heat and spray with cooking spray. Spoon pancake batter into the skillet. Cook until bubbles appear on the top and the edges look dry. Flip the pancake and cook until the bottom is golden brown.

Once all the pancakes are made, arrange on plates and serve each with a small handful of berries. Enjoy with a Metabolic Drive Low-Carb protein shake.

Serves 2

Chocolate Protein-Packed Cheerios
(Higher GI/GL)

    1 cup Cheerios
    1 cup skim milk
    1 scoop (20 grams protein) Chocolate Metabolic Drive
       Low-Carb

Pour the Cheerios into a bowl. In a blender or a shaker cup, mix the milk with the protein powder. Pour the mixture over the Cheerios.

Serves 1

Banana Breakfast Sandwich (Higher GI/GL)

    ⅓ cup egg whites (approximately 3 eggs)
    ¼ cup skim milk
    ½ teaspoon cinnamon
    2 large slices 12-grain or 100% whole-wheat bread
    1 medium ripe banana
    2 scoops (40 grams protein) Vanilla Metabolic Drive
       Low-Carb
    1 tablespoon honey

Preheat a nonstick skillet over low heat. In a medium bowl, whisk together the egg whites, milk, and cinnamon. Dip the bread into the mixture, coating both sides, and cook until golden brown, approximately 2 minutes on each side.

In a small bowl, mash the banana with a fork. Add the protein powder and honey and mix. Spread the banana mixture on one piece of toast, then top with the other piece of toast.

Serves 2

Apple-Carrot Muffins (Higher GI/GL)

Cooking spray

1 cup flour plus additional for dusting

1 teaspoon baking powder

1 large carrot

1 medium zucchini

5 scoops (100 grams protein) Vanilla Metabolic Drive
     Low-Carb

3 tablespoons true-to-measure Equal

1 cup unsweetened applesauce

1 tablespoon cinnamon

Preheat the oven to 350°F. Coat five cups of a muffin tin with nonstick cooking spray and dust with flour.

In a medium bowl, mix the 1 cup of flour and the baking powder. Grate the carrot and zucchini into another bowl. Add the protein powder, Equal, applesauce, and cinnamon to the carrots and zucchini. Fold in the flour mixture. Divide the mixture among the 5 muffin cups. Bake 30 to 40 minutes, or until a toothpick inserted in a muffin comes out clean.

Serves 5

Lumberjack's Breakfast (Higher GI/GL)

¾ cup yellow cornmeal

2 jalapeño peppers, seeded and chopped

2 tablespoons chopped parsley

2 tablespoons chopped green onions

½ cup nonfat plain yogurt

Salt to taste

⅔ cup egg whites at room temperature (approximately 5 eggs)

¼ teaspoon cream of tartar

Cooking spray

1 extra-lean 3-ounce turkey sausage

Preheat the oven to 350°F. In a small pot, boil the cornmeal with 1 cup of water until thick, approximately 15 minutes. Stir in the jalapeños, parsley, and green onions. Add the yogurt and a pinch of salt. Set aside.

Beat the egg whites with the cream of tartar until soft peaks form. Stir one-quarter of the egg whites into the cornmeal mixture, then gently fold in the remaining egg whites. Pour into a baking dish and bake until golden brown, about 45 minutes.

Spray a nonstick skillet with cooking spray and cook the sausage until golden brown on the outside and no pink is visible in the center. Serve with the bread.

Serves 2

Pumpkin Pancakes (Higher GI/GL)

1 cup pumpkin puree (pure pumpkin, not pumpkin pie
    filling)
1 teaspoon cinnamon
Pinch of nutmeg
1 scoop (20 grams protein) Vanilla Metabolic Drive
    Low-Carb
½ cup flour
2 teaspoons baking powder
Sugar-free maple syrup (optional)

Combine the pumpkin puree, cinnamon, nutmeg, and protein
powder in a small bowl. In another bowl, combine the flour and
baking powder. Fold the pumpkin mixture into the flour mixture.
If the mixture is too thick, thin with a little water.

Preheat a nonstick skillet over medium-high heat. Spoon the
batter into the skillet. Cook until bubbles appear on the top and
the edges look dry. Flip and cook until the second side is golden
brown. Top with sugar-free maple syrup if desired.

Serves 2

Turkey Polenta Cakes (Higher GI/GL)

2 3-ounce extra-lean turkey sausages
¾ cup cornmeal
Salt and pepper to taste
2 tablespoons low-fat plain yogurt
2 teaspoons chopped dill
1 to 2 dashes Tabasco

Preheat a nonstick skillet over medium heat. Slit one end of each sausage and squeeze its meat out from the casing. Cook until browned.

In a small pot, bring ⅔ cup of water to a boil and add the cornmeal. Cook, stirring constantly, for 10 to 15 minutes, or until thick. Its texture should be so that it can easily be formed into polenta cakes. Add water to thin if necessary.

Mix the turkey and polenta. Season with salt and pepper. Add the yogurt, dill, and Tabasco and mix well. Form into small patties and cook until golden brown, approximately 4 minutes on each side.

Serves 2

Banana-Yogurt Waffles (Higher GI/GL)

½ cup flour
2 teaspoons baking powder
1 scoop (20 grams protein) Vanilla Metabolic Drive Low-Carb
½ cup low-fat plain yogurt

½ cup skim milk

1 teaspoon vanilla extract

1 teaspoon grated lemon rind

1 medium ripe banana

Preheat a waffle maker. In a medium bowl, mix the flour, baking powder, and protein powder. Add the yogurt, milk, vanilla, and lemon rind. Mix well.

In a separate bowl, mash the banana with a fork and then add it to the flour mixture. Thin if needed by adding water, 1 teaspoon at a time.

Pour the batter into the waffle maker and cook according to the manufacturer's directions. (If you do not have a waffle maker, this recipe works well as pancakes.)

Serves 2

Protein Polenta with Bananas and Maple Syrup
(Higher GI/GL)

¾ cup skim milk

¾ cup cornmeal

2 scoops (40 grams protein) Vanilla Metabolic Drive Low-Carb

1 medium ripe banana, sliced

Sugar-free maple syrup

In a small pot, heat the milk over medium heat (do not boil). Add the cornmeal and cook, stirring, until thick, 10 to 15 minutes. Remove from the heat and cool. Stir in the protein powder. If the mixture seems too thick, thin with a little water. Divide between two bowls and top with the sliced banana. Drizzle with sugar-free maple syrup.

Serves 2

Roasted Potato Cheese Pie (Higher GI/GL)

4 new potatoes
½ teaspoon oregano
1 teaspoon rosemary
1 teaspoon garlic powder
Salt and pepper to taste
½ cup nonfat cottage cheese
¼ cup nonfat plain yogurt
½ cup chopped onions
3 drops jalapeño Tabasco sauce

Preheat the oven to 350°F. Cut the potato into small, thin fries. Place in a mixing bowl and toss with the oregano, rosemary, garlic powder, salt, and pepper. Place the potatoes on a baking sheet or in a roasting pan and bake for approximately 30 minutes, or until golden brown. Set aside to cool.

In a medium mixing bowl, combine the cottage cheese, yogurt, onions, and Tabasco. Add the roasted potatoes and mix well. Spread the mixture in a pie plate. Bake until the edges of the pie are golden brown.

Serves 2

Turkey Sausage Crepes (Higher GI/GL)

¾ cup flour

1 teaspoon vanilla extract

1 cup chopped mushrooms

1 garlic clove, minced

2 3-ounce extra-lean turkey sausages

1 tablespoon rosemary

2 tablespoons finely chopped chives

Salt to taste

Grated rind of ¼ lemon

1 tablespoon chopped mint

1 tablespoon chopped basil

Preheat a nonstick skillet over medium heat. In a mixing bowl, combine the flour, ⅔ cup of water, and the vanilla. Pour half the batter into the skillet and cook, flipping once, till both sides are golden brown. Set aside.

In the skillet, cook the mushrooms over low heat until most of their liquid has been released. Mix in the garlic, then add the sausage, rosemary, chives, and salt. When the sausage is browned, remove from the heat and slice the sausage. In a bowl, combine the sausage, lemon zest, mint, and basil.

Spoon half the sausage mixture onto half of each crepe, folding the remaining half over to cover.

Serves 2

Lunch Recipes

Filet of Sole with Black Olives and Feta Cheese
(Low Carb)

2 6-ounce sole filets

1 tablespoon olive oil

1 tablespoon lemon juice

Salt and pepper to taste

1 ounce feta cheese, crumbled

¼ cup sliced black olives

Preheat the grill or the oven to 350°F. Place each fish filet on a square of aluminum foil. Season the fish with the olive oil, lemon juice, salt, and pepper, then fold the remaining foil over to wrap each filet completely. Grill the foil-wrapped filets for approximately 15 minutes. Remove the fish from the foil and sprinkle with the feta cheese and olives.

Serves 2

Pork and Vegetable Stir-Fry (Low Carb)

8 ounces extra-lean pork tenderloin

1½ tablespoons olive oil

2 cups broccoli, chopped

1 red bell pepper, sliced

2 teaspoons soy sauce

¼ teaspoon red pepper flakes

3 tablespoons unsalted dry-roasted peanuts

2 tablespoons minced ginger

Trim any visible fat from the pork and cut the pork into slivers. Heat the olive oil in a nonstick skillet over medium heat. Stir-fry the meat for 5 minutes. Add the broccoli and bell pepper and cook for 2 minutes more. Add the soy sauce, pepper flakes, peanuts, and ginger and stir-fry for another 2 to 3 minutes.

Serves 2

Sliced Sirloin with Arugula and Feta Cheese
(Low Carb)

10 ounces extra-lean sirloin steak
Salt and pepper to taste
2 large handfuls of arugula
¼ cup sliced black olives
¼ cup feta cheese
Dash of lemon juice

Preheat the grill or a stovetop grill pan. Trim all excess fat from the steak. Season the meat with salt and pepper and grill for 5 minutes on each side for medium doneness.

Divide the arugula between two plates and top with the olives and feta cheese. Slice the steak and place on top of the arugula mixture. Sprinkle with lemon juice.

Serves 2

Spicy Chili-Rubbed Salmon with Grilled Zucchini (Low Carb)

1 tablespoon olive oil

1 tablespoon chili powder

¼ teaspoon cayenne pepper

9 ounces salmon filet

Salt and pepper to taste

1 garlic clove, minced

1 tablespoon rosemary

1 large zucchini, cut into wedges

Preheat the grill to medium-high. In a small dish, mix the olive oil with the chili powder and cayenne pepper. Rub the paste onto the salmon and season with salt and pepper. Place the salmon onto a large piece of aluminum foil and top with the garlic and rosemary. Add the zucchini. Fold up the edges of the foil to create "walls." Grill the fish until cooked through.

Serves 2

Grilled Tuna Salad (Low Carb)

8 ounces tuna steak

6 asparagus spears, trimmed

2 large handfuls of mixed greens

2 hard-boiled eggs

⅓ cup green olive slivers

1½ tablespoons olive oil

2 tablespoons balsamic vinegar

Juice of ½ lemon

Salt and pepper to taste

Preheat the grill to medium. Grill the tuna for 6 minutes, turning once. At the same time, grill the asparagus, turning frequently. Transfer to a cutting board and slice the tuna evenly into thin slices. Cut the asparagus into 1- to 2-inch chunks.

Divide the mixed greens between two plates. Crumble one egg over each plate and top with half of the olive slivers. Top the greens with the tuna and asparagus. Drizzle with the olive oil, vinegar, and lemon. Season with salt and pepper.

Serves 2

Salmon Kebabs and Green Beans (Low Carb)

10 ounces salmon, cubed

1 green bell pepper, cut into chunks

1 sweet onion, cut into chunks

2 cups green beans

Red wine vinegar to taste

Salt and pepper to taste

Lemon juice

Sesame seeds for garnish

Preheat the grill to medium. Skewer the salmon cubes, alternating with the pepper and onion. Grill for 8 to 10 minutes, turning every couple of minutes.

While the fish is cooking, cook the green beans in boiling water until slightly soft, about 5 minutes. Drain and put into a bowl. Add the vinegar, salt, and pepper and toss.

Arrange the skewers and green beans on two plates. Top with a squeeze of lemon juice and a sprinkle of sesame seeds.

Serves 2

Smoked Salmon with Dill Yogurt (Low Carb)

½ cup nonfat plain yogurt

¼ cup minced dill

2 cups bean sprouts

1 tablespoon olive oil

2 4-ounce pieces smoked salmon

Pepper to taste

In a small bowl, mix the yogurt and dill. Divide the sprouts between two plates and drizzle with the olive oil. Top each portion of sprouts with one portion of salmon. Season with pepper. Place a few spoonfuls of yogurt on each plate.

Serves 2

Swordfish with Steamed Green Beans (Low Carb)

¼ cup nonfat plain yogurt

1 teaspoon chopped green olives

1 tablespoon dry mustard

⅛ teaspoon store-bought seafood seasoning

½ tablespoon lemon juice

2 5-ounce swordfish steaks

2 cups green beans

Salt and pepper to taste

1 tablespoon olive oil

In a small bowl, combine the yogurt, olives, mustard, seasoning, and lemon juice and mix well. Allow to sit for at least a few hours in the fridge before serving, up to overnight.

Preheat the grill to medium-low. Grill the fish steaks just until the fish flakes at the touch of a fork, about 2½ minutes on each side. While the fish cooks, boil the beans in a small pot filled halfway with water until crisp-tender, about 3 minutes. Drain and divide between two plates. Add one piece of fish to each plate. Season with salt and pepper and drizzle with the olive oil. Top each piece of fish with 1 tablespoon of yogurt sauce.

Serves 2

Balsamic Chicken with Chickpea Puree
(Low GI/GL)

⅓ cup balsamic vinegar

½ cup chicken stock

2 garlic cloves, minced

2 medium chicken breasts

3 cups canned chickpeas, drained and rinsed

1 chicken bouillon cube

2 tablespoons chopped fresh thyme

Salt to taste

In a deep dish, combine the vinegar, chicken stock, and garlic. Marinate the chicken in this mixture for 20 minutes.

Preheat the broiler. Fill a small pot halfway with water and bring to a boil. Add the chickpeas and the bouillon cube. Boil for 5 to 7 minutes to soften the chickpeas. Drain the chickpeas, reserving the cooking water. Transfer the chickpeas to a blender with the thyme and salt and blend; adjust the consistency by adding 1 tablespoon at a time of the reserved cooking water until a smooth puree forms.

Put the chicken breasts in an oven-safe pan and broil for 12 to 15 minutes, or until done. Place some of the puree on each plate and top with a chicken breast.

Serves 2

Chicken with Roasted Onion and Mango Salad
(Low GI/GL)

2 medium skinless, boneless chicken breasts

Salt and pepper to taste

¼ teaspoon garlic powder

1 teaspoon olive oil

1 large red onion, sliced

2 large handfuls of mixed greens

1 large mango, sliced

2 lemon wedges

2 orange wedges

Preheat the grill to medium-high. Trim any excess fat from the chicken breasts. Season with salt, pepper, and garlic powder. Brush the grill with the olive oil to prevent sticking and grill the chicken, turning once, for approximately 5 minutes, or until done. While the chicken is cooking, grill the onion slices, flipping frequently, until browned.

Cool the chicken and onions for about 5 minutes. Place the greens into a salad bowl. Break the onion slices into rings and place them in the salad bowl. Add the mango. Squeeze the juice from the lemon and orange wedges over the salad and toss. Divide the salad between two plates. Slice the chicken breasts thinly and place on top of the salad.

Serves 2

Honey-Mustard Chicken Salad (Low GI/GL)

½ cup balsamic vinegar

3 to 4 tablespoons mustard

1 large garlic clove, minced

2 tablespoons honey

¼ to ⅓ teaspoon cayenne pepper

2 tablespoons olive oil

2 medium skinless, boneless chicken breasts

Salt to taste

1 white onion, diced

1 sweet red onion, diced

3 green onions, chopped

2 large handfuls of mixed greens

2 kiwis, sliced

Preheat the grill or a nonstick skillet over medium-high heat. In a small bowl, mix the vinegar, mustard, garlic, honey, cayenne pepper, and olive oil. Set the dressing aside.

Trim any excess fat from the chicken and salt both sides. Cook the chicken and onions for about 4 minutes, stirring the onions frequently. Turn the chicken and cook for another 4 minutes, or until done, while continuing to stir the onions.

Divide the greens between two plates. Slice the kiwi and divide between the plates. Slice the chicken and place on each salad. Top with the onions. Add the dressing and serve.

Serves 2

Warm Turkey Calzone (Low GI/GL)

7 ounces lean cooked turkey

3 hard-boiled eggs, whites only

½ cup chopped fresh basil

1 cup chopped sun-dried tomatoes

8 ounces 100% whole-wheat pizza dough, room temperature

Preheat the oven to 325°F. Cut the turkey into small pieces. In a medium bowl, crumble the egg whites. Add the basil, turkey, and tomatoes and mix well. Roll the dough into a square on a baking sheet. Place the filling at one end. Roll up and pinch the ends shut. Bake for 25 to 30 minutes, or until golden brown. Let sit for 10 minutes before serving.

Serves 2

Chicken Caesar Pita (Low GI/GL)

½ cup nonfat plain yogurt

1 tablespoon dry mustard

1 garlic clove, crushed

1 tablespoon anchovy paste

2 medium skinless, boneless chicken breasts

½ cucumber

1 100% whole-wheat pita

1 handful of romaine lettuce, shredded

Preheat the grill to medium. In a small bowl, mix the yogurt, mustard, garlic, and anchovy paste. Cook the chicken for about 3 minutes on each side. Slice the chicken and set aside.

Slice the cucumber into rounds. Cut the pita in half. Toss the lettuce, chicken, and cucumbers in a large bowl with the dressing. Divide the mixture between the two pita pockets.

Serves 2

Hamburger with Bean Puree (Low GI/GL)

8 ounces extra-lean ground beef

1 teaspoon chili powder

½ teaspoon garlic powder

Salt and pepper to taste

1 14-ounce can white beans, drained and rinsed

1 jalapeño pepper, seeded and sliced

5 or 6 mint leaves

1 teaspoon lemon zest

1 garlic clove

1 handful of fresh spinach

In a medium bowl, combine the meat, chili powder, garlic powder, salt, and pepper. Mix well with a fork or your hand. Form the meat into two patties. Pan-sear the burgers in a nonstick skillet over medium heat for about 10 minutes, turning once.

While the burgers cook, place the beans in a blender or food processor and add the jalapeño, mint, lemon zest, garlic, salt, and pepper. Puree until smooth.

Divide the spinach between two plates. Top with a burger and spoon the bean puree on top.

Serves 2

Tuna Steak with Olive Pesto (Low GI/GL)

¼ cup sliced olives

2 teaspoons olive oil

1 small garlic clove, minced

3 sprigs cilantro

1 teaspoon lemon zest

1 teaspoon red pepper flakes

2 4-ounce tuna steaks

½ cup baby spinach

2 100% whole-wheat buns

Place the olives, 1 teaspoon of the olive oil, the garlic, cilantro, lemon zest, and red pepper flakes in a blender and puree to a paste. Set aside.

In a nonstick skillet over medium heat, heat the remaining teaspoon of olive oil and sear the tuna for approximately 2 minutes on each side or until the desired doneness is reached. Arrange the spinach leaves on the buns and add the steaks. Top each with the pesto.

Serves 2

Asian Chicken Wraps (Higher GI/GL)

2 medium skinless, boneless chicken breasts

3 green onions, slivered

1 large carrot, slivered

2 tablespoons soy sauce

1 red chili, seeded and minced, or ¼ teaspoon red pepper flakes
    work just as well

1 tablespoon honey

2 100% whole-wheat tortillas

Sesame seeds

Cook the chicken any way you'd like—grilled, boiled, baked, or pan-seared. Cool the chicken and shred. Combine the chicken, green onions, and carrot in a medium bowl.

In a small bowl, mix the soy sauce, chili, and honey. Add to the chicken mixture and combine. Divide the chicken mixture between the tortillas, sprinkle with the sesame seeds, and roll up. Can be served warm or cold.

Serves 2

Hawaiian Baked Beans (Higher GI/GL)

3 cups (2 12-ounce cans) Bush's Original Baked Beans (or
    baked beans of your choice)
⅓ cup hickory smoke barbecue sauce
1½ cups diced fresh ham
1 cup diced pineapple, fresh or canned in juice, not syrup

In a medium pot, bring the baked beans in their sauce to a simmer. Reduce the heat to medium and stir in the barbecue sauce.
Add the ham and pineapple, mix well, and simmer for 10 minutes,
stirring occasionally.

Serves 4

Chicken Cacciatore Wraps (Higher GI/GL)

Cooking spray
1 white onion, thinly sliced
1 green bell pepper, thinly sliced
2 garlic cloves, minced
2 medium skinless, boneless chicken breasts
½ can tomato paste
3 canned plum tomatoes
Salt and pepper to taste
1 100% whole-wheat pita, halved

Preheat a large nonstick skillet over high heat. Coat the skillet
lightly with cooking spray and sauté the onion, bell pepper, and
garlic for 2 minutes. Add the chicken breasts and brown on both

sides. Add the tomato paste and tomatoes, crushing the tomatoes with a fork. Cook for approximately 10 minutes, or until the chicken is done. Season with salt and pepper. Divide the chicken mixture between the pita pockets.

Serves 2

Oven-Roasted Turkey and Cucumber Sandwich
(Higher GI/GL)

2 large slices 100% whole-wheat bread

Small handful of baby spinach

½ cucumber, thinly sliced

8 ounces lean oven-roasted turkey, sliced

½ small apple, cored and thinly sliced

Toast the bread. Arrange the spinach, cucumber, and turkey on one slice. Top the turkey with the apple slices and cover the sandwich with the remaining slice of bread. Cut in half.

Serves 2

Sirloin Steak with Peach-Cucumber Salsa and
Grilled Red Potatoes (Higher GI/GL)

3 peaches, pitted and sliced

½ cucumber, sliced

½ red bell pepper, thinly sliced

2 red potatoes, sliced

2 tablespoons rosemary

1 teaspoon garlic salt

10 ounces extra-lean sirloin

2 tablespoons lemon juice

Salt and pepper to taste

Preheat the grill to medium-high. Place the peaches, cucumber, and bell pepper in a medium bowl. Set aside. Season the potatoes with the rosemary and garlic salt.

Grill the steak for approximately 4 minutes on each side for medium doneness. While the steak is cooking, grill the potato slices for approximately 3 minutes on each side, or until slightly soft. Cut the potatoes into thin strips and add to the peach mixture. Add the lemon juice, salt, and pepper to taste and mix well. Serve alongside the steak.

Serves 2

BBQ Chicken Sandwich (Higher GI/GL)

7 ounces oven-roasted chicken breast

3 tablespoons barbecue sauce

½ cup diced red onions

8 ounces 100% whole-wheat pizza dough

Preheat the oven to 375°F. Tear the chicken into small pieces. In a small bowl, toss the chicken with the barbecue sauce and onion. Set aside.

Roll out the dough into a rectangle and place on a baking sheet.

Arrange the filling on one side and roll up the dough into a log shape, pinching the ends to seal and bringing the ends together to form a circle. Bake for 30 to 35 minutes, or until the bread is golden brown.

Serves 2

Variation: *Serve the chicken filling on 100% whole-wheat buns or bread.*

Oven-Roasted Chicken Breast with Roasted Pear Sandwich (Higher GI/GL)

1 Bosc pear, sliced thin
1 large handful of arugula
7 ounces oven-roasted chicken breast, cut into small pieces
2 tablespoons balsamic vinegar
1 large 100% whole-wheat pita, halved

Preheat the oven to 300°F. Place the pear slices on a parchment-covered baking sheet and bake until dried and golden brown. When the pears are cool, chop and toss them with the arugula, chicken, and balsamic vinegar. Divide between the pitas.

Serves 2

Rotis (Higher GI/GL)

8 ounces chicken breast
½ white onion, diced
½ cup green peas
1 garlic clove, minced
¼ cup white Minute Rice
½ cup nonfat plain yogurt
2 tablespoons curry powder
Salt and pepper to taste
2 100% whole-wheat tortillas

Preheat the oven to 300°F and heat a nonstick skillet over medium heat. Cut the chicken into bite-size pieces and cook in the skillet with the onion for 5 to 7 minutes, or until browned. Add the peas and garlic and cook for an additional 4 minutes.

Add the rice to the chicken mixture along with ½ cup of water. Bring to a boil and cook until most of the water has been absorbed. Add the yogurt and curry powder and mix well. Simmer until creamy. Season with salt and pepper.

Spoon equal portions into the tortillas and fold the tortillas over the filling, closing with a toothpick. Place onto a baking sheet and bake for approximately 10 minutes, or until golden brown.

Serves 2

Sun-Dried Tomato Pesto Pizza (Higher GI/GL)

2 cups sun-dried tomatoes

1 cup fresh basil

3 garlic cloves

1 to 2 tablespoons olive oil

8 ounces 100% whole-wheat pizza dough, room temperature

12 ounces nonfat cottage cheese

Preheat the oven to 400°F. Place the tomatoes, basil, and garlic in a blender and blend to a paste. Blend in the olive oil until the consistency is smooth enough to spread.

Roll the dough into a circle or rectangle and place on a nonstick baking sheet. Spread the pesto across the dough's surface. Top evenly with the cottage cheese and bake for 20 minutes, or until the edges of the dough are golden brown.

Serves 2

Dinner Recipes

Low-Carb Chicken Fajitas (Low Carb)

1 medium onion, chopped

2 medium bell peppers, cored, seeded, and chopped

1 tablespoon olive oil

1 pound chicken tenderloins, cut into thin strips
   lengthwise

1 packet fajita seasoning mix

4 Mission Carb Balance whole-wheat tortillas (fajita size)

1 cup reduced-fat shredded Cheddar cheese

In a skillet over medium heat, sauté the onion and peppers in the olive oil for 3 minutes. Add the chicken and cook for 10 minutes, or until done. Add the seasoning mix and ⅓ cup of water. Mix well, cover, and simmer for 5 to 7 minutes, stirring occasionally. Spoon onto the tortillas and top with the cheese.

Serves 4

Beer Can Chicken (Low Carb)

3 to 4 tablespoons tomato paste

2 to 3 tablespoons sugar-free honey

2 teaspoons cayenne pepper

1 tablespoon salt

1 teaspoon pepper

1 teaspoon garlic powder

Juice of ½ lime

½ onion, finely chopped

1 12-ounce can light beer

1 whole chicken

Olive oil

Preheat an outdoor grill to low. In a mixing bowl, combine the tomato paste, honey, cayenne pepper, salt, pepper, garlic powder, lime juice, onion, and beer and mix well. Do not discard the empty beer can. Rinse the chicken and trim any excess fat. Thoroughly rub the mixture all over the chicken, inside and out. (At this point you can leave the chicken in the refrigerator to marinate for 3 to 4 hours.) Insert the empty beer can into the chicken with the closed end facing out. Place a sturdy pan on the grill to catch the drippings. Stand the chicken on the pan so that it is resting on the beer can. Grill, covered, for about 1½ hours, checking frequently to make sure the chicken has not fallen over. When the chicken is fully cooked, remove the skin and serve with a light drizzle of olive oil on top.

Serves 4

Chicken with Arugula and Lemon Sauce (Low Carb)

4 medium boneless, skinless chicken breasts

Salt to taste

5 tablespoons olive oil

2 cups arugula

1 teaspoon black peppercorns

2 garlic cloves, smashed

1 tablespoon dried rosemary

Juice of 1 lemon

Grated zest of ½ lemon

½ cup dry white wine

Preheat a nonstick skillet over medium heat. Remove any visible fat from the chicken and salt both sides. Pour 2 tablespoons of the olive oil into the pan and heat for 10 seconds. Cook the chicken for 5 minutes on one side. Turn the chicken over and add the remaining 3 tablespoons of olive oil, the arugula, peppercorns, garlic, and rosemary. Cook for 2 to 3 minutes. Add the lemon juice and zest. Add the wine and cook for 6 to 7 minutes, then lower the heat and simmer for 3 minutes more.

Serves 4

Insalata Mista with Lemon-Garlic Chicken
(Low Carb)

1 garlic clove, minced

1 tablespoon dried rosemary

1 tablespoon chopped parsley

½ cup olive oil

½ cup white wine

Juice and grated rind of 1 lemon

Salt to taste

2 skinless, boneless chicken breasts

1 cup radicchio

1 cup arugula

1 cup spinach

⅓ cup white wine vinegar

⅓ cup olive oil

1 handful of fresh basil

In a small mixing bowl, combine the garlic, rosemary, parsley, ½ cup of olive oil, white wine, lemon juice, and lemon rind. Mix well and pour into a casserole dish. Salt both sides of the chicken breasts, place in the dish, turn to coat, and marinate in the refrigerator for 2 to 3 hours. One hour prior to cooking, remove the dish and place on the counter.

Preheat the grill to medium. Grill the chicken for 4 to 6 minutes on each side, until cooked through.

Chop or tear the radicchio, arugula, and spinach leaves and combine in a large bowl. In a blender or food processor, combine the vinegar, olive oil, salt, and basil and mix on low speed for 10 seconds. To serve, arrange the chicken breasts on plates accompanied by a portion of the salad. Drizzle on the desired amount of dressing.

Serves 2

Smoked Salmon with Portobello Mushrooms and Asparagus (Low Carb)

1 tablespoon minced parsley
1 tablespoon lemon juice
1 tablespoon olive oil
Portobello mushrooms—use desired amount
Asparagus—use desired amount
Salt and pepper to taste
10 ounces smoked salmon
1 tablespoon chopped fresh chives

Preheat an outdoor grill to medium. In a small bowl, combine the parsley, lemon juice, and olive oil. Grill the mushrooms and asparagus until tender and slightly charred. Arrange the vegetables on a plate and pour the oil mixture over them. Add salt and pepper. Place the salmon alongside the vegetables. Top everything with chives.

Serves 2

Sun-Dried Tomato Pesto Chicken (Low Carb)

2 cups sun-dried tomatoes
1 cup fresh basil leaves
1 to 2 garlic cloves, chopped
2 tablespoons grated Parmesan cheese
½ cup olive oil
4 medium skinless, boneless chicken breasts
Salt to taste

Preheat the oven to 350°F. In a blender or food processor, combine the tomatoes, basil, garlic, and cheese and mix on medium speed for about 5 seconds. Add the olive oil slowly and continue mixing on low speed for another 8 to 10 seconds. Butterfly the chicken breasts—thinly slice through the side of the breast without cutting all the way through (like cutting a roll or hot dog bun). Spread the pesto on one side of the opened chicken breast, then fold the other side on top to enclose the sauce. Sprinkle salt on top of the chicken. Wrap with cooking string or stick toothpicks through to secure. Set the chicken on a nonstick baking sheet and bake for 20 to 25 minutes, or until the chicken is fully cooked.

Serves 4

Chicken Souvlaki (Low Carb)

4 medium skinless, boneless chicken breasts, cubed

Salt and pepper to taste

½ cup nonfat plain yogurt

1 garlic clove, minced

1 tablespoon chopped fresh chives

½ white onion, grated

3 tablespoons olive oil

Preheat the grill to medium-high. Thread the chicken pieces onto skewers and season with salt and pepper. Cook, turning every 2 minutes, until the chicken is done. In a small bowl, combine the yogurt, garlic, chives, onion, and olive oil and mix well. Top the chicken with the yogurt sauce.

Serves 4

Haddock with Citrus-Chili Rub (Low Carb)

1 orange

1 lemon

4 5-ounce haddock filets

1 teaspoon brown sugar

3 tablespoons tomato paste

1 teaspoon chili powder

Salt and pepper to taste

4 tablespoons olive oil

2 handfuls of arugula

Grate the orange and lemon peel and set aside. Cut the orange and lemon into wedges and set aside. Lay the haddock filets skin side down in a glass casserole dish. In a small bowl, combine the brown sugar, tomato paste, grated orange and lemon rinds, chili powder, salt, and pepper and mix until it forms a paste. Rub the mixture on the top of each filet. Cover with plastic wrap and place in the refrigerator for 3 hours to marinate.

Preheat the oven to 350°F. Remove the plastic wrap from the dish and drizzle the olive oil over the fish. Add some lemon and orange slices alongside the filets. Bake, uncovered, until the fish flakes easily, 15 to 20 minutes. Serve with the arugula and remaining citrus slices.

Serves 4

Satay Chicken with Spicy Peanut Sauce
(Low Carb)

2 medium boneless, skinless chicken breasts, cubed

2 tablespoons olive oil

1 to 2 tablespoons all-natural peanut butter

1 teaspoon minced garlic

1 teaspoon cayenne pepper or to taste

1½ tablespoons lime juice

Salt to taste

Preheat the grill to medium. Skewer the chicken and brush with olive oil. Cook the chicken until done, turning every 2 minutes.

Bring the peanut butter and 1 cup of water to a boil in a small saucepan. Reduce the heat to a simmer. Add the garlic, cayenne pepper, lime juice, and salt and cook till thickened, about 5 minutes. Serve the sauce over the chicken.

Serves 2

Spicy Chicken and Roasted Pepper Salad
(Low Carb)

4 medium skinless, boneless chicken breasts

2 red bell peppers, sliced into thick strips

2 green bell peppers, sliced into thick strips

2 green onions, finely diced

3 garlic cloves, minced

½ cup minced parsley

1 teaspoon chili powder

1 tablespoon rosemary

6 tablespoons olive oil

Juice of ½ lemon

Preheat an outdoor grill to medium-high. Grill the chicken for 4 to 5 minutes on each side, or until done. While the chicken is cooking, grill the peppers until tender and lightly charred. Slice the cooked chicken into bite-size strips. In a large bowl, combine the sliced chicken, roasted peppers, green onions, garlic, parsley, chili powder, rosemary, olive oil, and lemon juice. Serve warm or cold.

Serves 4

Cheat to Lose Easy Chili (Low GI/GL)

1 pound extra-lean ground beef or turkey

1½ cups canned kidney beans

1½ cups canned pinto beans

1 16-ounce jar low-fat chunky garden-style tomato sauce

1 packet chili seasoning mix

In a large saucepan over medium heat, brown the beef. Stir in the kidney beans, pinto beans, tomato sauce, and chili seasoning. Bring to a boil, then reduce the heat, cover, and simmer, stirring occasionally, for 10 to 15 minutes.

Serves 4

Asparagus-Stuffed Chicken (Low GI/GL)

2 large skinless, boneless chicken breasts

Salt and pepper to taste

2 slices low-fat cheese, any kind

1 garlic clove, minced

1 teaspoon rosemary

Juice of ½ lemon

4 asparagus stalks, cut into halves

Preheat the oven to 350°F. Butterfly the chicken breasts (do not cut all the way through) and open flat. Season with salt and pepper. Lay the cheese on the bottom half of the opened filet. Add the garlic, rosemary, and lemon juice on top of the cheese.

Fill a small pot halfway with water and bring to a boil. Add the asparagus and cook for 1 to 2 minutes until soft. Drain and put four pieces of asparagus inside each opened filet. Fold the top part of the chicken over and secure with cooking string or toothpicks. Lightly spray a casserole dish with cooking spray and place the chicken in it. Bake for 35 to 45 minutes.

Serves 2

Caramelized Onions and Pork Chops (Low GI/GL)

4 4-ounce extra-lean pork chops
Salt and pepper to taste
1 white onion, chopped
1 green apple, chopped
4 tablespoons olive oil
2 tablespoons balsamic vinegar

Preheat the grill to medium-high. Season the pork chops with salt and pepper and grill for 5 to 7 minutes on each side, or until done.

In a nonstick skillet over medium heat, combine the onions, apples, and olive oil. Sauté just until soft, then lower the heat. Add the balsamic vinegar and cook for another 2 minutes, allowing the onions to caramelize. Serve over the pork chops.

Serves 4

Grilled Lean Pork with Peach-Mango Salsa
(Low GI/GL)

4 4-ounce lean pork chops

Salt to taste

2 mangoes, peeled, seeded, and diced

2 peaches, peeled, seeded, and diced

½ cup peeled and diced cucumber

¼ cup minced flat-leaf parsley

1 red chili pepper, minced, or 1 teaspoon red pepper flakes

2 tablespoons cider vinegar

½ tablespoon lemon juice

Pepper to taste

Preheat an outdoor grill to medium. Sprinkle the pork chops with salt and grill for 3 to 4 minutes on each side, until done. Combine the mangoes, peaches, cucumbers, parsley, chili pepper, vinegar, lemon juice, and pepper in a mixing bowl. Serve the salsa over or alongside the pork chops.

Serves 4

Shepherd's Pie (Low GI/GL)

1 pound lean ground turkey

4 cups mixed vegetables, fresh or frozen

1½ tablespoons rosemary

½ cup Dijon mustard

Salt and pepper to taste

¾ cup white wine

3 large sweet potatoes, peeled and cut into small chunks

1 teaspoon minced garlic

Preheat the oven to 350°F. In a large nonstick skillet, cook the turkey until brown, approximately 10 to 12 minutes. Add the vegetables, rosemary, mustard, salt, and pepper and mix well. Pour in the wine, lower the heat, and simmer for 5 to 7 minutes.

Boil the potatoes until soft. Drain the potatoes and return them to the emptied pot; add the garlic and mash.

Lightly coat a large baking dish with nonstick cooking spray. Pour the turkey and vegetable mixture into the dish, flattening it and packing it tightly. Spread the mashed sweet potatoes on top. Bake for 40 to 45 minutes.

Serves 4

Note: *Once assembled in the baking dish, this can be wrapped tightly and frozen up to 3 months. Simply remove from the freezer and uncover; place in a preheated 350°F oven and bake for 75 to 80 minutes.*

Bell Peppers Stuffed with Chicken and Whole-Grain Rice (Low GI/GL)

4 red or green bell peppers

½ cup whole-grain rice

2 cups frozen mixed vegetables

4 medium chicken breasts, cooked and chopped

Salt and pepper to taste

2 tablespoons olive oil

Preheat the oven to 350°F. Cut the tops off the peppers and remove the seeds and white ribs. Cook the rice and vegetables according to package instructions. Combine the rice, vegetables, and chicken in a bowl and season with salt and pepper. Pack the mixture into the peppers. Set the stuffed peppers in a casserole dish and drizzle the olive oil on top. Bake for 30 to 40 minutes.

Serves 4

Grilled Lamb and Couscous Salad (Low GI/GL)

1 cup couscous
1 medium zucchini, chopped
1 chili pepper, minced
4 green onions, diced
1 handful of mint leaves, minced
1 handful of coriander leaves, minced
Juice of 2 limes
Salt and pepper to taste
1 pound lean lamb tenderloin

Preheat the grill to medium. In a medium pot, bring 1 cup of water to a boil and add the couscous. Cook for 20 minutes, or until the couscous has absorbed all the water. Transfer the cooked couscous to a large bowl and combine with the zucchini, chili pepper, green onions, mint, coriander, lime juice, salt, and pepper. Grill the lamb for 3 to 4 minutes on each side, or until the desired doneness is reached. Slice the lamb into thin strips and serve on top of the couscous salad.

Serves 4

Lamb Chops with Beet-and-Orange Salad
(Low GI/GL)

5 tablespoons Worcestershire sauce

1 garlic clove, minced

1 tablespoon dried rosemary

Salt and pepper to taste

2 pounds lamb chops

2 large navel oranges, peeled and cut into bite-size pieces

3 cups sliced beets

5 green onions, chopped

¼ cup plus 1 tablespoon chopped parsley

1 cup plain nonfat yogurt

1 cup mint leaves, chopped

In a large bowl, whisk together the Worcestershire sauce, garlic, rosemary, salt, and pepper. Place the lamb chops in this mixture, turn to coat, and marinate for 1 hour in the refrigerator.

Preheat the grill to medium-high. In another large bowl, combine the oranges, beets, green onions, and ¼ cup parsley. In a separate bowl, combine the yogurt, 1 tablespoon parsley, and mint. Grill the lamb chops for 3 to 4 minutes on each side, or until the desired doneness is reached. Serve the lamb chops with the yogurt sauce.

Serves 4

Zucchini Parmigiana (Low GI/GL)

8 ounces extra-lean ground beef

½ onion, chopped

1 garlic clove, minced

1 28-ounce can diced or crushed tomatoes

½ cup minced parsley

Salt and pepper to taste

2 large zucchini

16 ounces nonfat cottage cheese

1 tablespoon olive oil

Preheat the oven to 350°F. In a skillet over medium heat, sauté the beef, onions, and garlic until the beef is no longer pink, 10 to 12 minutes. Add the tomatoes and bring to a boil. Reduce the heat, cover, and simmer for 10 minutes. Add the parsley, salt, and pepper and simmer, covered, another 10 minutes.

Slice the zucchini lengthwise into thin strips and lay on a paper towel to absorb some of the water. In a blender, puree the cottage cheese until smooth. Lightly coat a deep oven-safe dish with the olive oil. Place a layer of zucchini strips at the bottom of the dish, cover with some of the meat sauce, and then add a layer of cottage cheese. Continue to add layers in the same order until all the ingredients have been used. Cover the dish with aluminum foil and place in the oven. Bake for 15 minutes, remove the foil, and bake for another 10 minutes. Let stand for 5 minutes before serving.

Serves 4

Breaded Chicken with Rice (Higher GI/GL)

2 cups whole-wheat bread crumbs

2 tablespoons garlic salt

½ cup finely chopped flat-leaf parsley

3 tablespoons chopped rosemary

1 egg

½ cup egg whites (approximately 4 eggs)

4 medium boneless, skinless chicken breasts

1 tablespoon flour

2 cups whole-grain rice

1 lemon, cut into wedges

Preheat the oven to 400°F. In a small bowl, combine the bread crumbs, garlic salt, parsley, and rosemary. Transfer the mixture to a plate. In a separate bowl, whisk the egg and egg whites. Lightly dust the chicken with the flour. Dip the chicken into the eggs and then the bread crumbs. Place the chicken on a nonstick baking sheet and bake 15 to 20 minutes, until the bread crumbs are golden brown. While the chicken is baking, cook the rice according to package instructions. Serve the chicken over the rice with the lemon wedges on the side.

Serves 4

Green Pea Mashed Potatoes with Minced Beef (Higher GI/GL)

4 new potatoes, peeled and cut into small pieces

¾ cup canned peas

Salt and pepper to taste

8 ounces extra-lean ground beef

1½ cups sliced mushrooms

½ white onion, diced

1 cup chicken stock

¼ cup balsamic vinegar

1 teaspoon cornstarch

In a medium pot, cover the potatoes with water and bring to a boil over high heat. In a small pot over low-medium heat, heat the peas until boiling. When the potatoes are soft, drain, return them to the pot, and mash. Drain the cooked peas and puree them in a blender until smooth. Pour the peas into the potatoes, season with salt and pepper and mix well. Cover with a lid to keep warm.

In a nonstick skillet over medium heat, brown the beef. Drain the fat and set the meat aside. In the same skillet, sauté the mushrooms and onions until soft, 8 to 10 minutes. Add the beef back into the skillet. Pour the chicken stock over the beef and vegetables and simmer, uncovered, over medium heat for another 10 to 15 minutes. Add the balsamic vinegar and cornstarch, reduce the heat to low, and continue simmering until the sauce thickens, about 15 minutes.

Serves 2

Steak with Spicy Chili Cream and White Rice
(Higher GI/GL)

2 cups white rice

½ cup tomato paste

⅔ cup nonfat plain yogurt

1½ tablespoon chili powder

½ teaspoon cayenne pepper

12 ounces top beef round

½ white onion, diced

1 tablespoon olive oil

Prepare the rice according to package instructions. In a small bowl, combine the tomato paste and 1 teaspoon of water. Add the yogurt, chili powder, and cayenne pepper. Slice the beef into thin strips. In a nonstick skillet over medium heat, sauté the beef and onions with the olive oil for 10 to 12 minutes. Pour in the yogurt mixture and mix well. Cover and simmer for another 8 to 10 minutes. Serve the steak over the rice.

Serves 4

Turkey Pizza (Higher GI/GL)

¾ cup chopped red onion

1 garlic clove, minced

1 tablespoon olive oil

8 ounces extra-lean ground turkey

½ cup nonfat plain yogurt

¼ teaspoon cayenne pepper

2 100% whole-wheat pitas

1 28-ounce can diced tomatoes

¼ cup chopped parsley

Salt and pepper to taste

Preheat the oven to 450°F. In a skillet over medium heat, sauté the onion and garlic in the olive oil for 5 to 7 minutes, or until the onion is soft. Add the turkey and cook for another 10 to 12 minutes. Remove from the heat. In a bowl, combine the yogurt and cayenne pepper. Spread the yogurt onto each pita and add the turkey, then the tomatoes. Top with the parsley, salt, and pepper. Place in the oven and bake for 5 to 7 minutes, or until the pitas are crisp. Let the pizza stand for 5 minutes before serving.

Serves 2

Chicken Potpie (Higher GI/GL)

1 large boneless, skinless chicken breast
½ cup diced carrots
½ cup diced celery
½ cup drained canned corn
Salt and pepper to taste
8 ounces nonfat cottage cheese
8 ounces 100% whole-wheat pizza dough, at room
   temperature
¼ cup skim milk

Boil the chicken in water to cover for 5 to 7 minutes, or until cooked. Drain. When the chicken is cool enough to handle, cut into bite-size pieces and put into a large bowl. Add the carrots, celery, corn, salt, and pepper. Puree the cottage cheese in a blender until smooth, add to the chicken and vegetables, and mix well.

In a deep oven-safe baking dish, stretch the dough enough to cover the inside of the dish and have excess hanging over the sides. Pour the chicken and vegetable mixture into the dough shell and fold the edges over the filling. (It's fine if the dough does not reach the middle to fully cover.) Brush the dough with milk. Bake for 30 minutes, until the dough is light brown. Let the pie stand for at least 15 minutes before serving.

Serves 2

Sloppy Joes on 100% Whole-Wheat Buns
(Higher GI/GL)

1 pound extra-lean ground beef
1 white onion, finely chopped
½ cup tomato paste
¾ cup beef stock
¼ cup Worcestershire sauce
½ tablespoon chili powder
½ teaspoon cumin
½ teaspoon cayenne pepper (optional)
Salt to taste
4 100% whole-wheat buns

In a nonstick skillet over medium heat, sauté the beef and onion until browned, 10 to 12 minutes. In a bowl, combine the tomato paste, beef stock, Worcestershire sauce, chili powder, cumin, cayenne pepper, and salt. Pour the mixture over the beef and stir until well combined. Reduce the heat to low, cover, and simmer for 10 minutes. Warm the buns if desired, and split. Spoon the meat mixture over the buns.

Serves 4

Turkey Burger with Mixed Berry Sauce
(Higher GI/GL)

2 cups mixed berries

¼ cup raspberry vinegar

Juice of ½ lemon

1 pound extra-lean ground turkey

¼ cup finely diced sweet onion

1 tablespoon applesauce

¾ teaspoon cayenne pepper (optional)

Salt and pepper to taste

1 tablespoon whole-wheat bread crumbs

4 100% whole-wheat buns

Preheat the grill to medium. In a small bowl, combine the berries, vinegar, and lemon juice; set aside. In a large mixing bowl, combine the turkey, onions, applesauce, cayenne pepper, salt, and pepper and mix well. If the mixture is too moist, add the bread crumbs to thicken, 1 teaspoon at a time. Mold into 4 patties. Brush the grill with olive oil to prevent sticking and cook the burgers for 3 to 4 minutes on each side. Place each burger on the bottom half of a bun, top with the berry sauce, and cover with the other half of the bun.

Serves 4

Turkey Sausage with Potato Cakes (Higher GI/GL)

4 new potatoes

1 tablespoon plain low-fat yogurt

2 green onions, finely chopped

1 garlic clove

3 tablespoons finely chopped parsley

Salt and pepper to taste

2 3-ounce extra-lean turkey sausages, removed from casings

½ white onion, diced

½ cup frozen peas

2 tablespoons olive oil

Peel the potatoes and cut into small pieces. Heat a pot of water and boil the potatoes for 10 minutes or until soft, then drain, return to the pot, and mash. Add the yogurt, green onions, garlic, parsley, salt, and pepper and mix well. Cover and set aside.

In a nonstick skillet over medium heat, sauté the sausage, onions, and peas with 1 tablespoon of the olive oil until the sausage is fully cooked, 10 to 12 minutes, and transfer to a plate. Mold the potato mixture into patties. Add the remaining olive oil to the skillet and cook the patties until golden brown, 3 to 4 minutes on each side.

Serves 2

Protein Smoothie Recipes

Note: For all protein smoothie recipes, the use of a blender is recommended. Be sure to always place the liquid in the blender container first, then add the remaining ingredients one by one to ensure the smoothest final product. For a more milk-shake-like smoothie, add more ice.

Chocolate Mint Protein Smoothie

1½ scoops (30 grams protein) Chocolate Metabolic Drive
  Low-Carb
2 drops peppermint extract
1 cup cold water
4 ice cubes

For use on low-carb days. For low- or higher-GI/GL days, use 2 scoops Metabolic Drive Complete and 1 cup skim milk.

Chocolate Peanut Butter Protein Smoothie

1½ scoops (30 grams protein) Chocolate Metabolic Drive
  Low-Carb
2 tablespoons all-natural peanut butter
1 cup cold water
4 ice cubes

For use on low-carb days. For low- or higher-GI/GL days, use 2 scoops Metabolic Drive Complete and 1 cup skim milk.

Café Mocha Protein Smoothie

1½ scoops (30 grams protein) Chocolate Metabolic Drive
Low-Carb
1 teaspoon instant coffee
1 cup cold water
4 ice cubes

*For use on low-carb days. For low- or higher-GI/GL days, use 2 scoops
Metabolic Drive Complete and 1 cup skim milk.*

Pistachio Mint Protein Smoothie

1½ scoops (30 grams protein) Vanilla Metabolic Drive
Low-Carb
1 tablespoon sugar-free instant pistachio pudding
2 drops peppermint extract
1 cup cold water
4 ice cubes

*For use on low-carb days. For low- or higher-GI/GL days, use 2 scoops
Metabolic Drive Complete and 1 cup skim milk.*

Berry Blast Protein Smoothie

1½ scoops (30 grams protein) Vanilla or Strawberry Metabolic
   Drive Low-Carb
¼ cup fresh or frozen strawberries
¼ cup fresh or frozen blueberries
¼ cup fresh or frozen raspberries
1½ cups skim milk
4 ice cubes

For use on low- or higher-GI/GL days.

Apple-Cinnamon Oblivion Protein Smoothie

1½ scoops (30 grams protein) Vanilla Metabolic Drive Low-Carb
1 tablespoon sugar-free instant vanilla pudding (optional)
1 medium apple, cored and sliced into wedges
¼ teaspoon cinnamon
1 cup skim milk
4 ice cubes

For use on low- or higher-GI/GL days.

Peaches and Cream Protein Smoothie

1½ scoops (30 grams protein) Vanilla Metabolic Drive Low-Carb
1 tablespoon sugar-free instant vanilla pudding (optional)
1 peach, pitted and sliced into wedges, or the equivalent in
   frozen peaches
1 cup skim milk
4 ice cubes

For use on low- or higher-GI/GL days.

Cinnamon Bun Protein Smoothie

2 scoops Vanilla Metabolic Drive Complete
1 tablespoon sugar-free instant vanilla pudding (optional)
1 packet artificial sweetener
¼ teaspoon vanilla extract
¼ teaspoon cinnamon
¼ teaspoon nutmeg
1 cup skim milk
4 ice cubes

For use on low- or higher-GI/GL days.

Oats and Honey Protein Smoothie

2 scoops Vanilla Metabolic Drive Complete

½ cup (dry measurement) rolled oats cooked with water and cooled

1 tablespoon honey

1 cup skim milk

4 ice cubes

For use on low- or higher-GI/GL days.

Creamy Strawberry Passion Protein Smoothie

1½ scoops (30 grams protein) Strawberry Metabolic Drive Low-Carb

1 7-ounce container strawberry Dannon Light 'n Fit Yogurt Smoothie

½ cup fresh or frozen strawberries

1 cup skim milk

4 ice cubes

For use on low- or higher-GI/GL days.

Key Lime Pie Protein Smoothie

2 scoops Vanilla Metabolic Drive Complete

1 reduced-fat graham cracker, broken into pieces

1 tablespoon sugar-free instant vanilla pudding (optional)

1 tablespoon sweetened lime juice concentrate

1 packet artificial sweetener

1 cup skim milk

4 ice cubes

For use on higher-GI/GL days.

Strawberry-Banana Protein Smoothie

1½ scoops (30 grams protein) Strawberry Metabolic Drive
   Low-Carb

¼ cup fresh or frozen strawberries

1 ripe banana, peeled and broken into several pieces

1½ cups skim milk

4 ice cubes

For use on higher-GI/GL days.

Piña Colada Protein Smoothie

2 scoops Vanilla Metabolic Drive Complete

½ cup pineapple, fresh or canned in juice

1 tablespoon sugar-free instant vanilla pudding (optional)

¼ teaspoon coconut extract

1 packet artificial sweetener

1 cup skim milk

4 ice cubes

For use on higher-GI/GL days.

Chocolate-Banana Protein Smoothie

2 scoops Chocolate Metabolic Drive Complete

1 ripe banana, peeled and broken into several pieces

1 cup skim milk

4 ice cubes

For use on higher-GI/GL days.

Banana-Coconut Protein Smoothie

2 scoops Vanilla Metabolic Drive Complete

1 ripe banana, peeled and broken into several pieces

¼ teaspoon coconut extract

1 packet artificial sweetener

1 cup skim milk

4 ice cubes

For use on higher-GI/GL days.

Blueberry Cheesecake Protein Smoothie

1½ scoops (30 grams protein) Vanilla Metabolic Drive
   Low-Carb

1 reduced-fat graham cracker, broken into pieces

2 tablespoons no-bake, reduced-fat cheesecake mix

¼ cup fresh or frozen blueberries

1½ cups skim milk

4 ice cubes

For use on higher-GI/GL days.

S'mores Protein Smoothie

1½ scoops (30 grams protein) Chocolate Metabolic Drive
   Low-Carb
1 reduced-fat graham cracker, broken into pieces
2 tablespoons marshmallow cream
1 cup skim milk
4 ice cubes

For use on higher-GI/GL days.

Chocolate Lover's Protein Smoothie

2 scoops Chocolate Metabolic Drive Complete
1 packet fat-free hot cocoa mix
1 cup skim milk
4 ice cubes

For use on higher-GI/GL days.

Cookies and Cream Protein Smoothie

2 scoops Vanilla Metabolic Drive Complete

1 tablespoon sugar-free instant vanilla pudding (optional)

3 low-fat chocolate wafers

1 cup skim milk

4 ice cubes

For use on higher-GI/GL days.

Quick and Easy
Snack Recipes

Easy Low-Carb Protein Shake

1½ scoops Metabolic Drive Low-Carb
1 teaspoon fiber supplement
¾ tablespoon canola oil
1 cup cold water

Add the protein powder, fiber, and oil to water in a shaker cup and shake well.

Serves 1

For use on low-carb days.

Mixed Nut Beef Jerky Trail Mix

2 ounces beef jerky, broken into small pieces
Small handful of mixed nuts

Combine the jerky and nuts.

Serves 1

For use on low-carb days.

Chocolate Peanut Butter Protein Cookies

2 cups rolled oats

6 scoops (120 grams protein) Chocolate Metabolic Drive
   Low-Carb

2 12-ounce containers nonfat cottage cheese

¼ cup chunky all-natural peanut butter

Preheat the oven to 300°F. In a blender or food processor, grind the oats into a fine powder. In a large bowl, mix the oat flour, protein powder, cottage cheese, and peanut butter. Drop by ¼-cup portions onto a lightly greased baking sheet and bake for 12 to 14 minutes. Store refrigerated.

Makes 10 cookies, 2 cookies per serving

Variation: *To make vanilla-flavored cookies, use Vanilla Metabolic Drive Low-Carb and replace the peanut butter with 3 tablespoons canola oil.*

For use on either low- or higher-GI/GL days.

Berry Parfait

½ cup nonfat cottage cheese

4 ounces vanilla or strawberry Dannon Light 'n Fit Yogurt (or other nonfat, no-sugar-added yogurt)

1 scoop (20 grams protein) Vanilla or Strawberry Metabolic Drive Low-Carb

½ cup berries (blueberries, diced strawberries, raspberries, or blackberries)

⅛ cup low-fat granola

In a medium bowl, combine the cottage cheese and yogurt. Mix in the protein powder, a little at a time, until well incorporated. Top with the berries and granola.

Serves 1

For use on either low- or higher-GI/GL days.

Low-Carb Protein Pudding

½ cup nonfat cottage cheese

¾ tablespoon canola oil

1 scoop Metabolic Drive Low-Carb

Mix the cottage cheese well with the oil and protein powder. Add a little cold water at a time to thin if desired.

Serves 1

For use on low-carb days.

Peach Cobbler Parfait

½ cup nonfat cottage cheese

4 ounces vanilla Dannon Light 'n Fit Yogurt (or other nonfat, no-sugar-added yogurt)

1 scoop (20 grams protein) Vanilla Metabolic Drive Low-Carb

1 peach, peeled, pitted, and sliced

⅛ cup low-fat granola

In a medium bowl, combine the cottage cheese and yogurt. Mix in the protein powder, a little at a time, until well incorporated. Top with the peaches and granola.

Serves 1

For use on either low- or higher-GI/GL days.

Protein Pudding

⅓ cup skim milk

3 ice cubes

2 scoops Metabolic Drive Complete, any flavor

2 tablespoons sugar-free instant pudding, any flavor

Blend the skim milk and ice together on high, then reduce the speed to low. Remove the blender lid, and with the blender still on, add the protein powder and instant pudding mix little by little.

Serves 1

Tip: *Quadruple to prepare in bulk. Store refrigerated.*

For use on either low- or higher-GI/GL days.

Index